TREATMENT OF
COMMON ACUTE POISONINGS

Treatment of
Common Acute Poisonings

HENRY MATTHEW
M.D., F.R.C.P.Edin.

Physician-in-Charge, Regional Poisoning Treatment Centre,
Royal Infirmary, Edinburgh.
Director, Scottish Poisons Information Bureau.

ALEXANDER A. H. LAWSON
M.D., F.R.C.P.Edin.

Consultant Physician, West Fife Group of Hospitals

Foreword by
SIR DERRICK DUNLOP

THIRD EDITION

CHURCHILL LIVINGSTONE

EDINBURGH, LONDON AND NEW YORK

1975

CHURCHILL LIVINGSTONE
Medical Division of Longman Group Limited

Distributed in the United States of America by Longman Inc., New York and by associated companies, branches and representatives throughout the world.

© E. & S. Livingstone Limited, 1967.

© Longman Group Limited, 1975.

All rights reserved. No part of this publication may be reproduced, stored in a retrieval system, or transmitted in any form or by any means, electronic, mechanical, photocopying, recording or otherwise, without the prior permission of the publishers (Churchill Livingstone, 23 Ravelston Terrace, Edinburgh).

First Edition	.	.	.	.	1967
Second Edition	.	.	.	.	1970
Reprinted	.	.	.	.	1972
Third Edition	.	.	.	.	1975

ISBN 0 443 01217 2
Library of Congress Catalog Card Number 74-82390

Printed in Great Britain

FOREWORD

It is gratifying that my predictions of the success of this book which I made in writing the Foreword to its first edition have been so thoroughly justified. The three editions and a reprint published since 1967 amply testify to the popularity of its material and presentation.

It is a book about an important subject, for accidental poisoning and self-poisoning now constitute the most common cause but one for emergency admission to our general hospitals and is the most common cause of death but one among young people, especially girls, between the ages of 15 and 25. Self-poisoning is usually a preferable term to suicide, for the sub-conscious motive of most of those who poison themselves is to create a crisis providing an escape from some intolerable personal problem rather than actually to kill themselves. Nevertheless, they often succeed in doing so and the number of such deaths is beginning to approximate to that from road accidents. This epidemic of self-poisoning seems to be more common in welfare states than in countries where the primary concern of the population is the difficulty of securing sufficient food, clothing and shelter to keep alive. It corresponds with the increased use of hypnotics, tranquillisers, anti-depressants and mild analgesics. Such agents offer a more comfortable means of self-destruction than throat cutting, hanging or drowning. Further, it is simpler in some domestic crisis to draw attention to oneself by taking a handful of pills from the family medicine cupboard—so often replete with unused tablets of a psychotropic nature—than to develop an attack of the 'vapours' or crude hysteria which was a more common reaction in Victorian or Edwardian times. In addition, the ready availability and attractive presentation of modern medicines encourages the accidental poisoning of little children. It may be necessary in the future to ensure that tablets are invariably supplied in drug containers or reinforced plastic bubble packs which toddlers find very difficult to open. The trouble is that elderly people with arthritic hands may experience a similar difficulty.

The rapid advance of therapeutics—due largely to the ingenuity of the pharmaceutical industry—has made this new edition necessary rather than a further reprint: large numbers of potent, valuable but potentially dangerous new chemicals have been introduced in the last few years. Further, the pattern of self-poisoning has recently changed considerably. Barbiturates used to constitute 60 per cent of the agents used by poisoned adult patients admitted to hospital and salicylates 16 per cent. Barbiturates now only account for 20 per cent of such patients but there has been a corresponding rise in the incidence of poisoning by benzodiazepines such as chlordiazepoxide and diazepam and tricylic anti-depressants like amitryptaline and imipramine. With the considerable substitution of natural gas for coal gas the incidence of carbon monoxide poisoning has been much reduced. Salicylates continue to account for about 16 per cent of poisoned patients but in recent years, largely consequent on publicity given to it in coroners' courts, there has been an increase in self-poisoning by paracetamol—one of the safest of all effective drugs when used in therapeutic doses. Its dramatically successful recent treatment with cysteamine, described in this book, is most encouraging.

A qualified doctor is always expected to do something useful when faced with a medical emergency. This may be most embarrassing, for a medical degree does not necessarily confer on its possessor an invariable expertise in all such crises and his ignorance may cost lives. Every doctor should, therefore, possess a reference book of up-to-date treatment of acute poisoning. Such a book should concisely summarise the knowledge available, for in such emergencies it is most undesirable to have to consult voluminous texts. This is such a work—short, clear, dogmatic, easy of reference and concerned only with gross over-dosage and not with the side-effects of drugs (on which there are already a plethora of modern books) nor with reactions due to idiosyncracy in the patients.

Many works on toxicology are written by experts on forensic medicine, by pathologists, biochemists or public health officers, who may have little personal experience of treating poisoned patients, or by pharmacologists whose experience is confined to animals rather than to man. This book is written by physicians actively engaged in clinical medicine who treat their poisoned patients basically on much the same lines and by the same methods which they employ in their standard medical practice—seldom with antidotes but more often by eliminative procedures and by ordinary supportive measures such as the prevention of respiratory failure and the maintenance of a proper fluid and electrolyte balance. In recent years Dr. Matthew, Dr. Lawson and their colleagues have made the Poisoning Treatment Centre at the Royal Infirmary of Edinburgh and the associated Poisons Information Bureau famous; nor have they forgotten that the treatment of the somatic illness is often only a preliminary incident in the therapy of the tortured mind responsible for the emergency.

DERRICK DUNLOP

PREFACE TO THIRD EDITION

The management of acutely poisoned patients continues to be a rapidly increasing part of the work-load of busy acute medical units throughout the developed countries of the world. It is therefore all the more important to have a readily accessible and up to date manual of treatment for these patients, especially in view of the ever-increasing complexity of therapeutic agents used and the rising incidence of multiple drug overdoses taken. In this, the third edition of our book, we have made every effort to provide such a guide. For the sake of clarity and brevity, we have again adopted a rather dogmatic approach, but on th.s occasion we have provided a list of references for almost all the poisonings described in order that the reader may undertake further study of any of the subjects in which he may be interested.

We have considered carefully the many reviews of previous editions and from these and the evident demand, it seems reasonable to conclude that the presentation and composition of materials have met with general approval. However, with this edition we are endeavouring to reach an even wider readership. The basic style adopted in previous editions has been maintained but the third edition differs from its predecessors in a number of ways. The contents of several chapters have been rearranged and many poisonings have been brought under more general headings and so, although the number of poisonings described has been increased considerably and a more detailed text included, the total number of chapters has been reduced. The items contained in each chapter have been detailed in the list of 'contents' in order that the reader may easily see what the book contains.

Each chapter has been carefully revised and many have been extensively rewritten to take account of recent advances in treatment and changes in the pattern of toxic substances taken. The sections dealing with tricyclic drugs, paracetamol (acetaminophen), and paraquat have been greatly extended. Many poisonings have been added including propoxyphene, diphenoxylate, fenfluramine, oral hypoglycaemics, gold, thallium and poisonings due to venomous animals. In addition, where it was considered appropriate, proprietary preparations commonly used in the United States have been included.

Our thanks are due to the staff of Churchill Livingstone for their assistance and advice.

HENRY MATTHEW

Edinburgh, 1974   ALEXANDER A. H. LAWSON

PREFACE TO THE FIRST EDITION

In recent years the rising incidence of acute poisonings has become a considerable problem for all medical practitioners whether they work inside or outside hospital. A practical knowledge of the clinical features and the management of common acute poisonings is, therefore, essential.

This book has been based on our experience in the Poisoning Treatment Centre, Royal Infirmary, Edinburgh, and in the Scottish Poisons Information Bureau. It has been designed to provide practical advice on the common acute poisonings, which are described in detail. On the other hand, many time-honoured poisonings, such as arsenic, are in practice very uncommon and are described only briefly; others are not mentioned at all. Similarly, we have not provided an index of the numerous proprietary preparations. New products are introduced continuously and so any index arranged is almost immediately out of date. We have described the different poisonings under group headings, the advice given being, in some instances, applicable to a wide variety of different compounds. The ingredients of the great majority of currently prescribed preparations are listed in the generally available MIMS and Medindex, and further information is obtainable from the Poisons Information Service. The scope of the book is, therefore, intentionally limited and where a more detailed description is required the reader is referred to larger works.

In the last decade there have been many developments in the medical treatment of patients with acute poisoning. As a result, there has arisen a bewildering diversity of opinion regarding the most suitable and effective management. With due consideration of these various opinions, we have described here what we consider to be the safest, most practical and effective therapy for each poisoning. In particular, we have tried to indicate the uses and limitations of available methods to increase removal of poisons.

An essential part of the management of most of these patients is immediate psychiatric assessment and treatment. We have described the modern concepts of psychological disorder leading to self-administered poisonings. The psychiatric management and especially the social support required for these patients is also discussed in general terms.

Figure 2 is reprinted from the *British Medical Journal* (1965), **2**, 1269, by kind permission of Dr. Kessel and the *British Medical Journal*.

We thank Mrs. Mona Wilson, the publisher's editor, for much assistance and advice and we are particularly grateful to Dr. Stanley S. Brown for much helpful criticism.

HENRY MATTHEW
ALEXANDER A. H. LAWSON

Edinburgh, 1967

CONTENTS

CHAPTER   PAGE

1 INTRODUCTION 1
2 SIZE OF PROBLEM 4
3 POISONS INFORMATION SERVICE 10
4 DIAGNOSIS OF ACUTE POISONING 12
   Clinical—Visual identification—Laboratory identification.
5 BASIC PRINCIPLES OF MEDICAL TREATMENT . . . 17
   Milestones—Assessment of patient—Emergency measures—
   General care—Special care—Common errors in treatment.
6 SPECIAL METHODS OF TREATMENT OF INGESTANT POISONING 32
   Forced diuresis—Peritoneal dialysis—Haemodialysis.
7 BASIC PRINCIPLES OF PSYCHIATRIC TREATMENT . . . 43
8 ACUTE BARBITURATE POISONING 48
9 POISONING BY TOXIC INHALANTS 56
   Carbon monoxide—Kerosene and other petroleum distillates
   —Carbon tetrachloride—Cyanide—Benzene—Miscellaneous
   organic solvents.
10 ACUTE POISONING DUE TO COMMON ANALGESICS . . 69
   Salicylates—Phenacetin—Paracetamol (acetaminophen).
11 ACUTE POISONING WITH ANTIDEPRESSANT DRUGS . . 81
   Tricyclic compounds—Monoamine oxidase inhibitors—
   Lithium.
12 ACUTE POISONING WITH TRANQUILLISER DRUGS . . 89
   Phenothiazines—Rauwolfia alkaloids—Benzodiazepins—
   Carbamates—Meprobamate.
13 NON-BARBITURATE HYPNOTICS 97
   Glutethimide—Methaqualone—Chloral and its congeners—
   Ethchlorvynol.
14 NON-BARBITURATE ANTICONVULSANTS 105
   Hydantoin compounds—Paraldehyde—Sulthiame.
15 DRUGS WITH MAIN EFFECT ON AUTONOMIC NERVOUS
   SYSTEM 109
   Amphetamines — Fenfluramine — Ephedrine — Belladonna
   alkaloids.
16 ACUTE METALLIC POISONINGS 117
   Iron salts—Arsenic—Gold—Mercury—Lead—Phosphorus.
17 THE ALCOHOLS 128
   Methyl alcohol—Ethyl alcohol—Delirium tremens—Disulfiram.

18   DIGITALIS, QUININE AND QUINIDINE   134
19   OPIUM ALKALOIDS AND MORPHINE DERIVATIVES   .   .   138
     Opium and morphine—Propoxyphene—Diphenoxylate.
20   MISCELLANEOUS DRUGS   146
     Oral diuretics—Antihistamines—Oral anticoagulants—
     Contraceptive pills—Bromides—Thallium—Oral hypogly-
     caemic agents.
21   MISCELLANEOUS DOMESTIC AND INDUSTRIAL SUBSTANCES .   156
     Bleaches—Chlorate—Phenol, Lysol and Cresol—Naphtha-
     lene—Detergents—Metaldehyde—Turpentine—Matches.
22   VENOMOUS ANIMALS   163
     Snakebite—Insect bites—Venomous sea animals.
23   INSECTICIDES AND HERBICIDES   171
     Dinitro-ortho-cresol and dinitrophenol—Organophos-
     phorous compounds—Paraquat.
24   POISONOUS FUNGI, PLANTS, SHRUBS AND TREES   .   .   178
25   DRUG ADDICTION   184
     Stimulants—Depressants—Drugs causing distortion of the
     senses.
26   PREVENTION OF ACUTE POISONING   192

CHAPTER 1

INTRODUCTION

In recent years there has been a growing awareness in all the developed countries of the world, of the increasing incidence of acute poisoning. Accidental poisoning has increased, but the most significant rise has occurred in intentionally self-administered poisoning. The management of these patients places a considerable burden on the resources of doctors both inside and outside hospital practice.

Experience gained in the Regional Poisoning Treatment Centre, Edinburgh Royal Infirmary, and in the associated Scottish Poisons Information Bureau indicates that there are many misconceptions and fallacies regarding the treatment of patients with this condition. A successful outcome of the management in great measure depends on the efficiency and speed of emergency treatment. The purpose of this book is to provide a readily accessible and comprehensive guide to the management of acute poisoning, and to stress the basic principles of treatment. The regimens described are in general applicable to veterinary toxicology, especially regarding smaller animals.

In Edinburgh, there has developed over the last 100 years a centre providing special facilities for the medical treatment, toxicological investigation and psychiatric assessment of patients with acute poisoning, both accidental and otherwise. With this development general practitioners, ambulance drivers, nurses and even members of the general public in the surrounding area have come to recognise the unit as a district centre to which patients may be referred even when they are mildly poisoned. That this tradition is now firmly established is shown by the fact that about 90 per cent of all adult patients with acute poisoning, in a total population of approximately 750,000. are treated in the unit. The Regional Poisoning Treatment Centre admits patients above 12 years of age, but no younger children are treated.

For psychiatric considerations, it is the practice in the Centre, to admit all patients reported to be suffering from acute poisoning even when this is so mild as not even to be apparent. The work of the unit, therefore, provides an ideal opportunity to obtain statistical information on all aspects of poisoning. The statistics may be regarded as representative of the British population in general as there is no reason to suspect that Edinburgh people behave differently. In addition, since 1963 the staff of the Regional Poisoning Treatment Centre has manned the Scottish Poisons Information Bureau and this experience has provided valuable information regarding relevant problems and trends in other parts of Britain and further afield.

Since the design of this book has been based on these statistics the clinical features of the common poisonings due to barbiturates, salicylate, tranquillisers and anti-depressants are described in full, whereas the traditional but nowadays very uncommon intoxications, such as those due to arsenic or phenol derivatives are in general mentioned more briefly. There are some exceptions to this, such as cyanide poisoning, which is uncommon, but for which appropriate treatment must be given with great urgency. In such instances the emergency regime is detailed. It is hoped that in this way, appropriate practical information will be provided for the doctor faced with the problem of a patient who is suffering from acute poisoning.

Many doctors still labour under the illusion that for each poison there is a specific antidote. In practice, in less than 2 per cent of instances of poisoning is a true pharmacological antagonist available. In the vast majority of instances of poisoning, therefore, the treatment consists not in the application of the appropriate antidote, but in the employment of basic therapeutic principles to deal with symptoms and signs as they arise.

The basic principles of treatment which are described are, in the opinion of the authors, applicable equally to children and adults. There are, however, differences in the treatment of some specific poisonings, notably acute salicvlate overdosage, and in these cases significant variations where children are concerned are described.

Finally, it is important to note that the size of the overdose frequently bears little relationship to the severity of the underlying psychological disorder, and that treatment is therefore not completed with physical recovery of the patient. For this reason, a brief description of the present concepts of the psychiatric and social disorders which may lead to overdosage is included with a short discussion of the basic principles of the psychiatric assessment and initial management of poisoned patients.

CHAPTER 2

SIZE OF PROBLEM

Acute poisoning is now a common medical emergency often accounting for over 10 per cent of all acute adult medical admissions to most general hospitals [1-4]. The total annual mortality from poisoning has almost doubled in the past 14 years and in Britain nowadays almost equals that due to road accidents. Much dramatic propaganda is devoted to the prevention of death from road accidents and smoking, but little to the equally important prevention of fatalities from poisoning and gassing. Among the 25-34 year olds suicides constitute 1 in 10 of all deaths and in doctors death from suicide by poisoning is as common as death from carcinoma of lung[5, 6]. In children below the age of 10 acute poisoning is the fourth commonest cause of death, but this constitutes only 1 in 35,000 poisoning incidents. In adults, on the other hand, the mortality varies from 1-8 per cent of admissions to hospital[7].

The marked increase in the annual admission rate to the Regional Poisoning Treatment Centre of the Royal Infirmary, Edinburgh, is shown in Figure 1. The increase is a real one since there has been no change in admission policy over the years.

Acute poisoning may be classified as accidental, suicidal, homicidal or self-poisoning. 'Self-poisoning' is a conscious, often impulsive, manipulative act, undertaken to secure redress of an intolerable situation. It is in practice similar to what has been called 'attempted suicide' but is a wider concept which does not imply a particular motive. Thoughts of self-destruction are not prominent. In our experience accidental and suicidal poisoning each account for 10 per cent

4

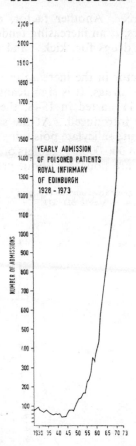

FIG. 1—Yearly admissions of poisoned patients, Royal Infirmary,
Edinburgh, 1928 onwards.

whereas 80 per cent indulge in self-poisoning. The major
reason for the large increase in admission of poisoned patients
to hospital is the marked rise in numbers of self-poisonings.
Accidental poisoning has also become more common but to a

much smaller degree. Another factor, especially in young adults and teenagers, is an increasing tendency in recent years for people to take drugs for 'kicks' and as a result of drug dependency[8].

An important factor in the increase of self-poisoning is the ready availability of drugs. It is significant that the sharp rise in incidence (Fig. 1) started in 1948, the year the National Health Service was introduced. At the same time, however, the incidence of acute salicylate poisoning also started to rise, but over half of the 4,000,000,000 tablets of salicylate consumed annually in Britain are bought without prescription.

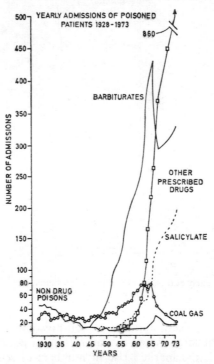

Fig. 2—The changing pattern of poisonings over the years.

CHANGE IN CHIEF DRUG INVOLVED

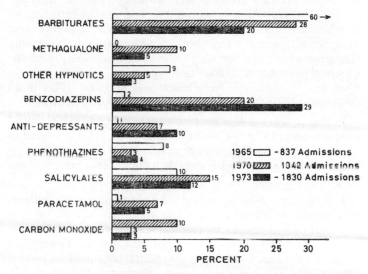

FIG. 3—Change in chief drug involved.

Acute poisoning is commonest between the ages of 16 and 25; in this group the female to male ratio is 3:1. In the age group 40-49 years, it is approximately two females to one male and beyond this age the incidence is equal in both sexes[6]. In Edinburgh, one in every 1,000 adults and one in every 600 teenage girls annually indulges in self-poisoning. Elsewhere in Britain one in every 100 married teenage girls behaves in this manner.

Different forms of poisoning predominate in each age group. The teenager rarely gasses herself, preferring to take salicylate; the reverse is true with older patients.

Fashions in the choice of drug have changed over the years (Figs. 2 and 3). An important feature demonstrated is that the recent fall in acute barbiturate poisoning has been more than compensated by a continued increase in poisoning by other prescribed drugs. 'Other prescribed drugs' include the non-barbiturate hypnotics, tranquillisers and antidepressants, all of which are prescribed so liberally for the very patients most likely to indulge in self-poisoning. In contrast to the increasing frequency of overdosage with these drugs, poisoning with the group of substances called 'non-ingestants', such as arsenic, lysol, etc., has become very much less popular. This is no doubt related to the ready availability of hypnotic drugs.

In recent years it has become common practice for several different drugs to be taken at the same time. This occurred in 26 per cent of our admissions. Alcohol is also involved to some extent in over 50 per cent of male patients and in about 25 per cent of females.

It is important to note that all acutely poisoned patients will require psychiatric help and that they should not be regarded with antipathy by medical staff or nursing attendants in spite of the self-imposed nature of their illness. Twenty-five per cent will require in-patient psychiatric treatment; a further 40 per cent will need out-patient psychiatric follow-up; 15 per cent require follow-up by psychiatric or other social workers. Only 20 per cent require no psychiatric treatment. As many as 36 per cent of patients repeat the self-poisoning within one year. Although some of these repeaters are psychopaths, for whom little can be done, Kennedy[9] has shown that in Edinburgh, if patients with poisoning are treated at home, they are three times more likely to repeat the act than those admitted to hospital.

It will be seen therefore that acute poisoning is nowadays a very real medical and social problem in developed countries. It is not isolated to any geographic or social group and so it must concern every practising doctor. In particular, self-poisoning, which has become a recognised pattern of social behaviour, is a crisis situation which must be treated as such with the maximum effort from medical, psychiatric and social welfare services.

REFERENCES

1 World Health Organisation (1968). *Wld. Hlth. Organ. techn. Publ. Hlth. Paper*, **35.**

2 Matthew, H., Proudfoot, A. T., Brown, S. S. and Aitken, R. C. B. (1969). *Brit. med. J.*, **3,** 489.

3 Sydney Smith, J. and Davidson, K. (1971). *Brit. med. J.*, **4,** 412.

4 Lawson, A. A. H. and Mitchell, I. (1972). *Brit. med. J.*, **4,** 153.

5 Lester, D. (1970). *Soc. Psychiat.*, **5,** 175.

6 Kennedy, P., Kreitman, N. and Ovenstone, I. M. K. (1974). *Brit. J. Psychiat.*, **124,** 36.

7 Reid, D. H. S. (1970). *Arch. Dis. Childhood*, **45,** 428.

8 Forrest, J. A. H. and Tarala, R. A. (1973). *Brit. med. J.*, **4,** 136.

9 Kennedy, P. (1972). *Brit. med. J.*, **4,** 255.

CHAPTER 3

POISONS INFORMATION SERVICE

The first telephone service giving information on poisons was established in Chicago in 1953 and called a Poisons Control Centre. Since then most developed countries have organized some form of Poisons Information Service.

Specific information on poisons has been available in Britain since a telephone service first started in Leeds in 1961. The Health Authorities in Britain established an official information service in 1963. Centres were set up in Belfast, Cardiff, Edinburgh[1] and London, the service being co-ordinated from the Centre located in London[2]. The aim is to provide a service to doctors who may wish to enquire by telephone whether a substance, often ingested by a child, is poisonous and if so what treatment is advised. It was considered that this service should be available only to doctors, as the information contained in the Bureau is frequently of a confidential nature, and as it was felt that only a doctor on the spot could adequately assess the implications of the information given in relation to the patient. A physician is always available at each of these Centres to provide information and discuss the management of a poisoned patient. It is, however, always stressed that the responsibility for treatment must remain with the doctor in charge of the patient.

The Centres have available information on the nature and toxic effects of some 10,000 substances used in the home, agriculture, industry and medicine. The number of enquiries both from general practitioners and hospitals is steadily increasing each year.

Emphasis is placed on providing the essential information as briefly as possible. This contrasts with comparable services

TABLE I

TELEPHONE NUMBERS OF POISONS INFORMATION SERVICE

Government sponsored	
BELFAST	0232-40503
CARDIFF	0222-33101
DUBLIN	Eire Dublin 45588
EDINBURGH	031-229-2477
LONDON	01-407-7600
LEEDS	0532-32799
MANCHESTER	061-740-2254

in Europe, North America and Australasia where a vast
amount of data is usually given to the enquirer, who may be
a member of the public. In the United States there are 580
Poison Control Centres[3, 4].

REFERENCES

1 Matthew, H. (1973). *Hlth. Bull.*, **31**, 1.
2 Goulding, R. (1971). *Hlth. Bull.*, **29**, 170.
3 Verhulst, H. L. and Crotty, J. J. (1971). Poisons Information Service
   and Barbiturate Poisoning. In *Acute Barbiturate Poisoning*, Ed.
   Matthew, H., p. 313. Excerpta Medica Monograph. Amsterdam:
   Excerpta Medica.
4 National Clearinghouse for Poison Control Centers, U.S.A. (1971).
   Bulletin Nov.-Dec.

B

CHAPTER 4

DIAGNOSIS OF ACUTE POISONING

Often the circumstantial evidence may be so strong that there is no doubt that a patient has taken poison. This is particularly the case in patients with self-poisoning who, before becoming drowsy or losing consciousness, intimate what has been done. It may also be equally evident in the determined suicide who takes elaborate precautions to avoid premature discovery and leaves a suicide note.

It should be remembered that poisoning may occur quite apart from ingestion or inhalation. Some toxic substances such as weed-killers and certain insecticides may be readily absorbed through the skin. Toxic chemicals in industrial use may be readily absorbed percutaneously and acute salicylate poisoning has occurred from the use of salicylic acid ointment on extensive skin lesions.

Few poisons produce diagnostic features. The smell of coal gas makes this diagnosis self-evident. Pin-point pupils, vomiting, depressed respiration and loss of consciousness may be helpful in the diagnosis of poisoning by morphine and related alkaloids. Flushing, sweating, tinnitus, deafness, tachycardia and over-breathing strongly suggest acute salicylate poisoning. Dull white burns of the buccal mucosa and grey burns of the lips and the chin indicate poisoning with caustic or corrosive substances; the smell of lysol is characteristic of intoxication due to phenol derivatives. The finding of blisters on the skin, often on an area of erythema, strongly suggests barbiturate as the cause of coma. These lesions occur in 6 per cent of patients with acute barbiturate poisoning[1]. They are found most commonly in sites where pressure has been exerted between two skin surfaces such as the interdigital clefts and inner aspects of the knees: they are seldom seen in areas of maximum pressure. Bullae may occur in other acute poisonings, notably glutethimide, tricylic antidepressants, methaqualone, meprobamate and carbon monoxide[2].

The combination of hypertonicity, exaggerated limb reflexes often with clonus, extensor plantar responses and myoclonia in addition to an impaired level of consciousness favours a diagnosis of Mandrax (methaqualone and diphen-hydramine) poisoning. Loss of consciousness with widely dilated pupils, bladder distension, absent bowel sounds, cardiac arrhythmias and prominent features of pyramidal tract involvement are frequently associated with overdosage by tricylic compounds.

It is as well to remember that in the age group 15-50, apart from head injury, the commonest cause of impaired consciousness is acute poisoning and even in older patients this diagnosis must be considered.

VISUAL IDENTIFICATION

It is our strong belief that the emergency management of these patients must be based primarily on a clinical assessment and that it is dangerous if efforts to identify the poison result in a delay in resuscitation. Therefore valuable time should not be lost in attempting to identify such substances at the outset, but confirmation of the types of poisoning should subsequently be made as patients now commonly take more than one poison at the same time. Identification of poisons may be also of medico-legal and epidemiological importance.

An increasing number of tablets can be readily recognised by markings imprinted on their surface or by their characteristic shape or colour. Many manufacturers now imprint the name of the drug house on the tablet or capsule and at the same time supply coloured illustrations of their products. Such charts may be of assistance in identification but colour fading presents a real problem. The marking of tablets and capsules with a code letter and number has recently been introduced and is of assistance.

The recommendations of the British Pharmacopoeia Commission that the colouring of tablets of official preparations is to be discouraged has led to the manufacture of a vast number of uncoated tablets. These uncoated tablets vary in shape and size, and these characteristics are used in the method of identification devised by McArdle[3].

In America the scheme described by Hefferren[4] in which size, colour, shape and markings are listed has proved of value. However, it is important to remember that even with the best methods of physical identification, the empty bottle found beside the patient or brought to hospital may not be the one from which the tablets or fluid were taken. It has even happened that the capsules clutched in the hand of an unconscious patient were not, in fact, the remnants of what had been consumed.

LABORATORY IDENTIFICATION

Qualitative identification of a substance in gastric aspirate, blood or urine will provide a definitive diagnosis of poisoning. Chemical analysis of most poisons requires elaborate laboratory equipment and specialised technique. The recent trend is for an increasing number of patients to take complex overdoses of different drugs and the clinical assessment of these patients may be aided by toxicological studies. The value of ward side-room tests, therefore, has become limited except for salicylate which may be estimated by a modification of the method of Trinder[5, 6].

Principle of the Method

Salicylate reacts with ferric iron to form a purple coloured complex. The intensity of this colour, which is proportional to the salicylate concentration up to approximately 100 mg per 100 ml, is measured by comparison with a series of Lovibond permanent glass colour standards. Mercuric chloride and hydrochloric acid are used to precipitate the plasma proteins.

The Standard Lovibond Comparator Disc 5/41

This disc contains nine standards corresponding to 15, 25, 35, 45, 55, 65, 80, 95 and 110 mg of salicylic acid per 100 ml of plasma (Note 1).

Technique

To 0·5 ml of plasma (Note 2) in a 12·5 mm diameter disposable tube add 5 ml of Trinder's reagent. Stopper and mix well by shaking vigorously: allow the tube to stand for five minutes. Centrifuge for five minutes and then place the tube in the right-hand compartment of the comparator with a blank prepared from 0·5 ml of water and 5 ml of the reagent in a tube in the left-hand compartment. Stand the comparator in front of a standard source of white light, such as the Lovibond White Light Equipment or, failing this, north daylight and match the colour of the supernatant liquid in the tube with the standards in the disc.

Notes

1. The common symptoms of salicylate poisoning are generally considered to be evident when plasma levels exceed 30 mg per 100 ml. It is unusual to find patients with levels higher than 80 mg per 100 ml; in such cases, the assay should be repeated with 0·25 ml of plasma, 0·25 ml of water and 5 ml of reagent, and the result multiplied by two to give the plasma level.

2. Heparin should be used as the anticoagulant for the original blood sample; oxalate or citrate is not suitable. High levels of bilirubin, of glucose or of urea, or a slight degree of haemolysis do not affect the salicylate reading.

The methods of estimation of other common poisons require more specialised knowledge and expertise. The more important of these are described in the following:

Technical Bulletin of Annals of Clinical Biochemistry, No. 24 (1972), **9**, 35.

Clarke, E. G. C. (1969). *Isolation and Identification of Drugs*. London: The Pharmaceutical Press.

Curry, A. (1969). *Poison Detection in Human Organs.* 2nd ed. Springfield: Charles Thomas.

Sunshine, I. (1969). *Handbook of Analytical Toxicology.* Cleveland: C. R. C. Press.

Curry, A. (1972). *Advances in Forensic and Clinical Toxicology.* Cleveland: C. R. C. Press.

In general laboratory identification of the poison taken is of more immediate value than the quantitative determination of the blood or urine level, which may be misleading as a guide to the severity of the intoxication. The reason for this is that there is such a wide individual variation in response to drugs, that published fatal blood levels can only indicate the general order of toxicity of a given drug. For example, patients with epilepsy who have developed tolerance to phenobarbitone may be only slightly drowsy with blood levels well above the suggested potentially fatal level, whereas those who are not habituated in this way may be deeply comatose and dangerously ill at blood levels well below this. The management and prognosis of these two types of patient are entirely different. This obtains with any drug to which tissue tolerance can be achieved and the liver microsomal enzyme system has been stimulated. Many drugs may share the same metabolic pathway and so in situations of enzyme system alert the drug effects may be considerably lessened.

REFERENCES

1   Beveridge, G., and Lawson, A. A. H. (1965). *Brit. med. J.,* **1,** 835.
2   Matthew, H. (1972). *Lancet,* **2,** 874.
3   McArdle, C. and Skew, E. A. (1961). *Lancet,* **2,** 924.
4   Hefferen, J. J. (1962). *J. Am. med. Ass.,* **182,** 1146
5   Trinder, P. (1954). *Biochem. J.,* **57,** 301.
6   Brown, S. S. and Smith, A. C. A. (1968). *Brit. med. J.,* **4,** 327.

CHAPTER 5

BASIC PRINCIPLES OF MEDICAL TREATMENT

Acute poisoning has been shown to be very common. It is, therefore, important that every doctor should have a considered regimen of management for these patients.

In the course of the last 25 years there have been very important advances in treatment. It is of value to consider briefly the history of various regimens of therapy using acute barbiturate poisoning as a model. In 1945 (Fig. 4) no fewer

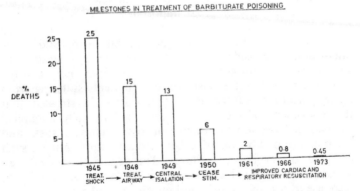

MILESTONES IN TREATMENT OF BARBITURATE POISONING

FIG. 4—Milestones in the treatment of barbiturate poisoning.

than 25 per cent of all patients with this form of overdosage died. With improved methods for the treatment of shock and for the maintenance of respiration, this mortality was reduced to 10-15 per cent. The next major advance followed the introduction in Copenhagen of a specialised unit for the treatment of acute poisoning. As a result of this centralisation

17

Clemmesen was able, within one year, to reduce the mortality by one half; finally, by avoiding analeptic treatment, a mortality of only 2 per cent was achieved. This successful regimen of management has become generally known as the Scandinavian method[1]. Considerable modifications of this treatment have been developed as a result of experience gained in the Regional Poisoning Treatment Centre, Edinburgh, where the mortality from acute barbiturate poisoning is less than 0·5 per cent[2].

INTENSIVE SUPPORTIVE THERAPY

This regimen consists of (a) assessment of the patient, (b) emergency measures, (c) general care and (d) special care.

Assessment of Patient

When a doctor first sees a patient with acute poisoning, the initial assessment is of great importance, not only to gain a baseline estimation of the patient's condition by which subsequent progress may be judged, but also, and more important, to consider the need for emergency measures to support vital functions. There is very confusing advice in the literature regarding the assessment of patients suffering from acute poisoning. It cannot be too strongly stressed that the assessment of the patient must be primarily a clinical assessment based on the degree of loss of consciousness and the presence or absence of other medical complications, such as shock or respiratory failure. The degree of loss of consciousness is assessed according to the response or lack of response to painful stimuli, and may be graded as:—

Grade I.   Drowsy but responds to vocal command.
Grade II.   Unconscious but responds to minimal stimuli.
Grade III. Unconscious and responds only to maximal painful stimuli.
Grade IV.   Unconscious and no response whatsoever.

The standard painful stimulus is rubbing the patient's sternum with the clenched fist. Contrary to general belief the size and activity of the pupils and the state of the limb reflexes are too variable to be useful indices of the severity of the poisoning. Absence of bowel sounds on auscultation of the abdomen is often associated with grade III, and nearly always with grade IV unconsciousness.

Other schemes [3, 4] have attempted to include the patient's overall clinical state in addition to depression of consciousness, but we consider these to be too complicated to be of practical value.

It is frequently suggested that the levels of poison in circulating blood are of vital importance in assessing patients, and some even attempt to indicate varying degrees of severity according to these levels. For the reasons already given (p 16) this is not in general satisfactory. Some patients may be very deeply unconscious with a blood level of 2·0 mg/100 ml of sodium amytal, whereas others, who have become habituated to the same drug, may be ambulant at levels of 8·0 mg/100 ml. Apart from diagnostic purposes, the measurement of such levels is almost valueless in the assessment of patients. Important exceptions to this rule are found in acute salicylate poisoning where the clinical picture in adults may be very deceptive; in such cases the assessment of the severity of the poisoning should take into account measurement of plasma levels of salicylate. Another exception is acute paracetamol poisoning.

Emergency Measures

These may be discussed under three sub-headings:
1. Respiratory failure.
2. 'Shock'.
3. Prevention of further absorption of poison.

Respiratory Failure

This is a common complication of acute overdosage due to sedative drugs, and emergency measures to correct it are frequently required. It is absolutely essential to maintain a clear airway[2]. After removing debris from the mouth and fauces the patient should at all times be nursed on his side to avoid the ever present danger of inhalation of vomit or secretions. It is most important that any unconscious patient must be kept in this position during transportation to hospital. A very frequent error is that the patient is placed on his back during the journey by ambulance to the hospital. This is a common cause of aspiration pneumonia which is an important factor in morbidity and even mortality. Suffocation may occur. An oropharyngeal or cuffed endotracheal tube, depending on the grade of unconsciousness, should be inserted. The cuff is inflated by introducing about 5·0 ml of air into the side tube on the airway. An objective measure of respiratory function may be obtained using a Wright's spirometer. This instrument, although not highly accurate, especially at low flow rates, which is a disadvantage in children, is nevertheless sufficiently so for practical purposes, and has the great advantage of being simple to use[3]. If the minute volume is less than 4 litres, significant respiratory depression should be assumed and arterial blood taken for measurement of pH, Pco_2, standard bicarbonate and Po_2. On the basis of these findings, further appropriate treatment may be given. If the Po_2 is reduced but above 60 mm Hg and the Pco_2 lies between 40 and 50 mm Hg, oxygen therapy should be administered using initially a 24 per cent Ventimask (oxygen flow rate 4·0 litres per minute). The arterial blood gases should be repeated after 30 minutes and if there is no further rise in Pco_2 a 28 per cent Ventimask should be used. Careful and continued monitoring of the arterial blood gases is necessary until the patient's condition becomes satisfactory.

Respiratory failure is present if the Po_2 falls below 60 mm Hg and, or the Pco_2 is greater than 50 mm Hg[4]. Hand ventilation using a Water's canister should then be given for 30 minutes. If improvement in the arterial blood gases is not sustained after a further 30 minutes of treatment, artificial respiration using a mechanical respirator will be necessary. Occasionally, in extreme cases, it may be necessary to give 2·0 ml nikethamide (Coramine) in order to stimulate respiration temporarily, while other measures to support respiratory function are being prepared. Provided the above regimen is followed, analeptic drugs to stimulate the respiratory centre will not otherwise be needed. Tracheostomy is seldom necessary and should never be performed unless endotracheal intubation is still required after 48 hours[5, 6]. However, with plastic tubes the risk of tracheal damage and subsequent stenosis is reduced and intubation can be continued safely for several days longer.

Shock

There is debate about what constitutes shock, but in practice it may be assumed to be present if the systolic blood pressure falls below 90 mm of mercury in a patient over 50 years of age, and below 80 mm in a younger patient. However, measurement of the central venous pressure, when facilities are available, will provide a more accurate means of monitoring the effective circulation of patients.

In recent years the mechanism of shock, particularly in acute barbiturate overdosage, has been extensively studied[8, 9]. There is evidence that apart from central cardiac depression, the main causative factor is a reduction in cardiac output resulting from diminution of the circulating blood volume. This relative hypovolaemia is the result of an increased capillary permeability with loss of fluid to the extracellular space; there also appears to be marked venous pooling, particularly in the lower limbs where there is considered to be incompetence of the venous valves. All these mechanisms operate to produce a net reduction in the venous return to the heart. It is probable that similar mechanisms operate in the shock associated with other sedative drugs. From these considerations it would seem logical to give intravenous infusions to re-establish the circulating blood volume. In practice, however, the authors have found that if elevation of the lower limbs is ineffective in raising the blood pressure, intravenous doses of 2·5 mg of metaraminol (Aramine) at 20 minute intervals should be given. The aim is to elevate the systolic blood pressure to no more than 100 mm of mercury, since above this level, metaraminol produces a net reduction in cardiac output and intense vasoconstriction of the renal arterioles, with great danger of resultant renal damage. If two, or possibly three, consecutive injections of metaraminol fail this treatment should be abandoned and plasma expanders such as low molecular weight dextran or plasma itself should be used. Oxygen therapy is indicated in all patients in whom there is a sustained fall in blood pressure. Arrhythmias should be corrected by appropriate drugs and digitalis and diuretics given where there is congestive cardiac failure. Acidaemia, which may contribute to the shock, should be sought by measurement of the arterial blood pH and, if present, treated by infusion of bicarbonate. In resistant cases, hydrocortisone (100 mg) intravenously and repeated at six hourly intervals may be of value. It is important to remember, however, that steroids delay the metabolism of barbiturates, thus prolonging recovery.

The regimen of metaraminol already described is both very simple and very satisfactory, without any significant complications provided the appropriate precautions are taken. It should be noted also that although the circulatory blood volume is diminished, these patients are seldom dehydrated— quite the contrary; they have tissue fluid excess. If the circulating blood volume is therefore reconstituted in the stage of severe poisoning it is possible that, with reversal of the above defects during the period of recovery, the patient may suffer acute circulatory embarrassment. This is particularly likely in the older patients in whom the cardiotoxic and vascular effects of drugs may be more marked.

Prevention of Further Absorption of the Poison

This is the third emergency measure. It may be achieved by inducing vomiting or performing gastric lavage. The ingestion of paraffin, kerosene and similar petroleum distillates is a contraindication to this measure (p. 63). In view of the danger of inhaling gastric content, vomiting should only be induced when a conscious patient is lying on his side with the head dependent. Children should be placed in the 'spanking' position. The best method of inducing vomiting is still the traditional one of irritating the pharynx with the finger or a blunt spoon-handle. The popular use of salt solutions, especially in children, may cause acute electrolyte disturbance and is best avoided. Emetic drugs, such as apomorphine, are dangerous in effective dosage as they may induce protracted vomiting and shock and are not recommended. These harmful effects can, however, be overcome by an injection of naloxone (p. 140). Syrup of ipecacuanha has been enthusiastically advocated, but this also cannot be generally recommended, as the emetic effect is often too slow and even if vomiting does occur, emptying of the stomach is usually incomplete. In addition, in circumstances when vomiting does not occur the emetine content of the ipecacuanha may be absorbed and itself produce toxic effects. Finally if the patient should become drowsy before the emetic effect is produced there is a considerable hazard of inhalation should vomiting subsequently occur. Copper preparations were employed with increasing frequency as emetics in children. They do not appear to be any more effective than syrup of ipecacuanha and are not recommended as they are too toxic. Activated charcoal administered orally can effectively reduce the absorption of salicylate, barbiturate, glutethimide, propoxyphene, ethchlorvynol and kerosene. However, it also inactivates syrup of ipecacuanha and so the two should not be given together[10]. Oral cholestyramine has been shown also to reduce paracetamol absorption[11].

In hospital, provided the patient has an adequate cough reflex or is sufficiently unconscious to permit cuffed endotracheal intubation, and the lungs thereby protected, gastric aspiration and lavage should be undertaken if there is evidence that the drug has been swallowed within the previous four hours[12]. After that interval, it is unlikely that there will be any worthwhile recovery of the ingested poison, except with salicylate and tricyclic preparations which may be recovered many hours after ingestion. The aspirate and an aliquot of

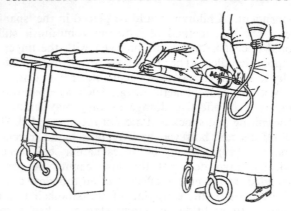

FIG. 5—Position of patient.

the lavage fluid should be kept for chemical analysis.

All too often these valuable procedures are incorrectly performed. The position of the patient is most important (Fig. 5). It is essential that the patient be placed in the head down position and turned on his left side, and kept thus throughout the procedure. Although technically simple, there is always the danger of aspiration and suction apparatus must be immediately available at all times. The correct equipment is also vital (Fig. 6). An adequate size of tube such as a 30 English gauge Jacques tube passed through the mouth must be used. This is of sufficient bore to make it extremely unlikely that the tube will enter the patient's trachea, and it permits removal of semi-solid food particles. Although this tube is large it is, in practice, very easy to insert and, therefore, is less upsetting to the patient than smaller tubes. Once the tube is securely in the stomach, aspiration is performed using a Dakin's syringe. Lavage is then carried out with 300 ml portions of warm water (38°C) and continued until the recovered fluid is clear. This may require at least 40 l of lavage fluid. In children appropriate sizes of tubes and volumes of water should, of course, be used. Except in

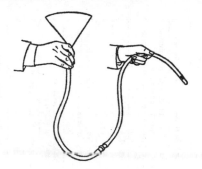

FIG. 6—Apparatus for gastric lavage.

the specific instances shown in Table II there is no need to use any other form of fluid and nothing should be left in the stomach at the end of the procedure. The so called 'universal antidote' which is sometimes used in gastric lavage is certainly not an antidote and is itself dangerous on account of its tannic acid content.

General Care

This includes nursing care, correction of water and electrolyte balance and acid-base status. Hypothermia may also require specific treatment.

Nursing Care

This must be of a high order. A successful outcome largely depends on the skill and application of the nurses in the positioning and regular half-hourly turning of the patients to prevent the occurrence of pressure sores. On each occasion when the unconscious patient is turned full passive movements of all limbs and percussion of the chest, followed by suction of the upper respiratory tract and endotracheal tube must be performed with great thoroughness to prevent blockage. Half-hourly estimations of the pulse, blood pressure, temperature and level of consciousness are also

TABLE II

OCCASIONS WHEN THE LAVAGE FLUID SHOULD BE OTHER THAN WARM WATER AND THE VARIOUS SUBSTANCES WHICH SHOULD BE LEFT IN THE STOMACH ON COMPLETION OF LAVAGE. IT IS IMPORTANT, HOWEVER, TO NOTE THAT FURTHER IMMEDIATE TREATMENT SHOULD NOT BE DELAYED WHILE THE SUBSTANCES RECOMMENDED ARE BEING PREPARED.

Poisoning	Lavage fluid	Substances left in stomach at end of lavage
CYANIDE	25 per cent sodium thiosulphate	200 ml. of freshly made mixture of two solutions: (a) 6 per cent sodium carbonate; (b) 15·8 per cent ferrous sulphate in 3 per cent citric acid.
IRON	2 g. desferrioxamine to 1 litre of warm water.	5 g. desferrioxamine in 50 ml. water.
GLUTETHIMIDE (Doriden)	Equal quantities water and castor oil.	50 ml. castor oil.
OPIATE	Dilute potassium permanganate. One solution-tablet (B.P.C.) dissolved in 3¾ litres (6 pints) of warm water.	Nil. Make sure potassium permanganate has all been removed by lavage with warm water.
BLEACH (containing sodium hypochlorite)	2·5 per cent sodium thiosulphate.	50 ml. of milk of magnesia or 100 ml. 2·5 per cent sodium thiosulphate.
OXALIC ACID	1 per cent calcium gluconate.	100 ml. 1 per cent calcium gluconate.
PHENOL, CRESOL, LYSOL	Mixture of 2 to 1 warm water and castor oil.	50 ml. castor oil.
PHOSPHORUS	0·1 per cent copper sulphate in water.	50 ml. of 0·1 per cent copper sulphate in water.

required. In seriously ill patients cardiac and respiratory monitoring is highly desirable. When bullous lesions are present on the skin (p. 12) and these may be quite extensive, they should be treated in the same way as superficial burns. The roof of each blister should be removed with appropriate sterile precautions and every effort made to prevent the area becoming infected. If this is achieved, these lesions will heal without scarring as they are intra-epidermal. Particularly when these lesions occur on the fingers and toes the patient may experience numbness and paraestheslae in the areas. These symptoms may persist for some time, but the patient should be reassured that they will eventually resolve spontaneously.

Water and Electrolyte Balance

Dehydration should be treated in the same way as in any other situation of fluid and electrolyte loss. If the patient can drink and is not vomiting, oral fluids will be sufficient to effect rehydration. When this is not possible, intravenous infusions of 1,000 ml of 5·0 per cent dextrose and 500 ml of normal saline in rotation are usually sufficient, the rate of infusion depending on the patient's condition. There may on occasion be severe changes in acid-base status and in plasma electrolytes. Correction of these abnormalities requires adequate biochemical support.

Hypothermia

A subnormal temperature is also a common finding. When the rectal temperature is below 36° C the patient may be said to be significantly hypothermic. Low-reading rectal thermometers are an essential part of the equipment of any intensive care unit and should be used whenever there is the slightest suspicion that the patient might have a low body temperature. If this is not checked even marked hypothermia might be undetected, with serious consequences. In general active reheating should be avoided, and all that is necessary is to prevent further heat loss by nursing in a warm room at approximately 26° C[13] and wrapping the patient in foil. If the hypothermia is marked or prolonged, hydrocortisone (100 mg) intravenously should be given at six hourly intervals. Hypoglycaemia may require correction.

Occasionally severe hypothermia, with a rectal temperature of less than 29·5° C is found. In this circumstance metabolism becomes sluggish and the body tends to behave rather like an inanimate object, and so further heat loss is likely to continue. In such cases active reheating is necessary. The patient should be insulated with blankets and the forearm immersed in a warm water bath at 43° C[14]. A rise in body temperature of 4°C per hour may be anticipated but if this treatment fails peritoneal dialysis or the administration of warmed oxygen by a modified Waters anaesthetic circuit[15] may be life-saving. A mini-coil artificial kidney may also be used to warm perfused blood.

Common Errors in Treatment

There are common, important misconceptions in treatment. The main ones concern analeptic therapy, intravenous infusion, bladder catheterisation, and prophylactic antibiotics.

Analeptic Therapy

Bemegride (Megimide) and other analeptic drugs are often given. Bemegride is not a specific barbiturate antagonist and has no part to play in the treatment of this form of poisoning; nor should analeptics be used in the treatment of poisoning by other sedative or hypnotic drugs[16, 17]. The only indication for analeptic therapy is the use of nikethamide in an emergency as a respiratory stimulant to maintain the patient whilst more adequate measures to support respiration are being prepared (p. 20). As already noted (Fig. 4, p. 17) when analeptic drugs were in vogue for treating barbiturate poisoning, the overall results were very disappointing, and the available statistics indicated a mortality of about 20 per cent. This was attributed to the complications of the treatment, particularly cardiac arrhythmias and convulsions, which may produce cerebral ischaemia and depression or even irreversible brain damage. Visual hallucinations and psychoses have also been reported after bemegride dosage. The 'awakening effect' of these drugs is, moreover, only transient and they are generally ineffective in severe poisoning.

Bemegride in plasma interferes with some commonly used methods of estimation of barbiturate and glutethimide.

Intravenous Infusion

In the absence of dehydration, it is unnecessary to give parenteral fluids for the maintenance of fluid and electrolyte balance in the first 12 hours even in unconscious patients.

Bladder Catheterisation

Generally speaking the dangerous procedure of bladder catheterisation is unnecessary even in deeply unconscious patients and incontinence of urine usually means in fact that a patient will soon recover consciousness. On the other hand it is undesirable to leave a grossly distended bladder and, if simple hand pressure does not readily provoke a urine flow, catheterisation is necessary. Otherwise, it is required only in exceptional situations when special methods to hasten elimination of the poison are used and the maintenance of an accurate fluid balance is important.

Prophylactic Antibiotics

Provided there is sufficiently intensive toilet of the mouth and airway together with half-hourly turning and physiotherapy, routine prophylactic antibiotics to prevent respiratory infection are not required[18]. Indeed on general principles they are contraindicated. Antibiotic therapy should, therefore, be reserved for the situation where there is clear clinical or radiological evidence of infection.

Poisoning Due to Noxious Gases

The regimen described so far has been directed towards acute poisoning due to ingestants. The basic principles of supportive therapy to maintain vital functions apply equally well to inhaled gases as to poisons taken by mouth, but a few additional comments are required.

It is obvious that the most immediate step must be to remove the patient into a fresh atmosphere. As the main effect of the poison is initially likely to be on the respiratory system, measures to support respiration are often very urgently required. Artificial respiration must be given immediately if indicated, and if possible oxygen therapy begun. Mouth to mouth breathing should be avoided. Nikethamide (2·0 ml) intravenously may be required as an emergency measure. If there is severe bronchospasm, aminophylline (0·5 g) intravenously is required. If there are marked pulmonary secretions frusemide (Lasix) 40 mg should be given intravenously. When the secretions are due to the irritant effects of certain noxious gases, hydrocortisone (100 mg) intravenously at six-hourly intervals over the first 24 hours after exposure is of value. In severe cases oxygen therapy should be given according to the results of arterial blood gas analysis.

Summary

When the Scandinavian method of supportive therapy was first introduced it was heavily criticised as being a regimen of 'therapeutic nihilism'. The intensive supportive therapy described here, which is an important development from that regimen, is far from being nihilistic and, on the contrary, to be successful demands the most intensive nursing and medical care. That this treatment is highly successful in Edinburgh is shown by the results of a survey of its use in 10,134 patients.

TABLE III

1967-1973—METHODS TO INCREASE ELIMINATION IN 10,134 PATIENTS

Forced Diuresis	308*
Peritoneal Dialysis	7
Haemodialysis	10

*266 suffering from salicylate poisoning.

Intensive supportive therapy was found to be adequate in over 97 per cent of patients, the remaining 3 per cent requiring in addition more specialised techniques of treatment (Table III).

REFERENCES

1 Clemmensen, C. and Nilssen, E. (1961).   *Clin. Pharmacol. Ther.*, **2**, 220.

2 Lawson, A. A. H. and Proudfoot, A. T. (1971).   Medical management of acute barbiturate poisoning.   In *Acute Barbiturate Poisoning*, ed Matthew, H., p. 175.   Excerpta Medica Monograph.   Amsterdam: Excerpta Medica

3 Reed, C. E., Driggs, M. F. and Foote, C. C. (1952),   *Ann. Intern. Med.*, **37**, 290.

4 Baker, A. B. (1969).   *Med. J. Aust.*, **1**, 497.

5 Sykes, M. K., McNicol, M. W. and Campbell, E. J. M. (1969).   *Respiratory Failure*, p. 211.   Oxford: Blackwell.

6 Tonkin, J. P. and Harrison, G. A. (1966).   *Med. J. Aust.*, **2**, 581.

7 Lindholm, C. E. (1969).   *Acta anaesth. scand.*, *Suppl.* 33.

8 Shubin, H. and Weil, M. H. (1965).   *Am. J. Med.*, **38**, 853.

9 Shubin, H. and Weil, M. H. (1971).   Shock associated with barbiturate intoxication.   In *Acute Barbiturate Poisoning*, ed. Matthew, H., p. 135.   Excerpta Medica Monograph.   Amsterdam: Excerpta Medica.

10 Leader (1972).   *Brit. med. J.*, **3**, 487.

11 Dordoni, B., Willson, R. A., Thompson, R. P. H. and Williams, R. (1973).   *Brit. med. J.*, **3**, 86.

12 Matthew, H., Mackintosh, T. F., Tompsett, S. L. and Cameron, J. C. (1966).   *Brit. med. J.*, **1**, 1333.

13 Hockaday, T. D. R. (1969).   *Brit. J. hosp. Med.*, **2**, 1083.

14 Cooper, K. E. (1968).   Temperature regulation and its disorders.   In *Recent Advances in Medicine*, ed. Baron, D. N. *et al*, p. 333.   London: Churchill.

15 Lloyd, E. L. (1973).   *Brit. J. Anaesth.*, **45**, 41.

16 Myschetzky, A. (1961).   *Dan. med. Bull.*, **8**, 33.

17 Montani, S. and Perret, C. (1963).   *Schweiz med. Wschr.*, **93**, 692.

18 Hadden, J., Johnson, K., Smith, S., Price, L. and Giardina, E. (1969).   *J. Am. med. Ass.*, **209**, 893.

CHAPTER 6

SPECIAL METHODS OF TREATMENT OF INGESTANT POISONING

In recent years several techniques have been developed which are considered to promote removal of various poisons from the body[1]. There has been an unfortunate trend to use these methods much too readily. It has been suggested that patients who are merely drowsy should be subjected to such treatment without critically assessing whether the procedure will, in fact, increase elimination or whether the patient will not regain consciousness satisfactorily with intensive supportive therapy alone. The natural process of recovery sometimes receives scant attention. Consideration is not given as to whether the patient is tolerant, habituated or addicted to the drug taken in overdosage, in which event he is likely to regain consciousness sooner than would be the case in a patient who has not been exposed to the noxious agent. Neither are the dangers inherent in the method of treatment assessed.

There is at present no way of predicting how long an individual patient will remain unconscious. Claims that a particular form of treatment has shortened the period of unconsciousness are therefore not valid[2]. Studies with control series are misleading for even the same patient does not necessarily behave in a predictable way on repeating the same overdose. Claims that certain amounts of drug have been recovered during a form of treatment may also be misleading for according to the method of assay a large proportion of the recovered 'drug' may represent inactive metabolites. Studies of blood levels of drugs can also give rise to misunderstanding. As already stated, the epileptic, tolerant to pheno-

32

barbitone, may be awake with a serum level of 10 mg per cent whereas another patient will be deeply unconscious at the same serum level. Such levels in the context of assessing severity of poisoning are largely meaningless.

Much research, therefore, requires to be undertaken before methods attempting to increase elimination of a particular drug can be regarded as properly evaluated and their place in treatment established. Acute salicylate poisoning has been studied in this way and forced alkaline diuresis is established as an effective form of therapy for overdosage of this particular drug.

The methods by which attempts may be made to increase elimination of poisons include:
1. Forced diuresis using various regimens[3, 4].
2. Peritoneal dialysis[5, 6, 7].
3. Extracorporeal dialysis[2, 4].
4. Exchange transfusion[8].
5. Passage of blood over ion exchange resins or other adsorbing material[9].

Each of these methods is not without its own risks, especially when used in severely ill patients. It is important to appreciate the basic requirements that must obtain if a given method is to be successful in removing a particular poison.

Forced Diuresis
The greater the amount of unchanged or pharmacologically active form of the drug excreted by the kidney, the greater will be the success of this method.

Contraindications to the Use of Forced Diuresis
1. Knowledge that the poison in its active form is not excreted by the kidney.
2. Shock.
3. Cardiovascular decompensation.
4. Impaired renal function.

5. Production by poison of pulmonary oedema.
6. Lack of facilities to monitor plasma electrolyte levels, except in salicylate poisoning.

Forced 'Cocktail' Diuresis for Acute Salicylate Poisoning Technique

1. Saline,   0·9 per cent — 0·5 litre
   Dextrose   5 per cent   — 1 litre
   Sodium bicarbonate   1·26 per cent — 0·5 litre
   Potassium chloride   3 g

   given as a mixture at a rate of 2 litres per hour for three hours and thereafter 1 litre per hour until the serum salicylate is less than 35 mg per cent when the drip may be stopped.

   The rate of infusion is most important.

2. Copious fluid intake by mouth as soon as the patient can tolerate this.

3. Bladder emptied hourly.

Pulse respiration and blood pressure should be charted every half hour. The fluid intake and output must be accurately recorded.

The rate of infusion in young children is 30 ml/kg/hour and monitoring of the plasma potassium and other electrolytes is important in children.

Precautions

1. If an adult patient is drowsy in the absence of accompanying sedative drug overdose, acidaemia should be suspected and corrected by prior infusion of 500 ml of 5 per cent sodium bicarbonate within 30 minutes prior to the start of the above regimen.

2. The regimen is subject to the patient maintaining a normal jugular venous pressure and to the absence of signs of pulmonary congestion.

Forced Alkaline Diuresis

Technique

Intravenous infusion of:

0·9 per cent saline
5·0 per cent dextrose   } 500 ml in rotation.
1·26 per cent sodium bicarbonate

Intravenous K^+ supplements (1 g KCl) should be added to each 500 ml bottle from the sixth bottle in the infusion regime. These fluids must be given at a rate of 2 litres per hour for three hours and 500 ml thereafter. Mannitol 5 per cent and frusemide may be added.

Adjustments in the regimen may have to be made according to the patient's response and fluid and electrolyte balance. Careful biochemical monitoring is essential.

The urinary pH should be measured hourly and, if below 7·5, substitute 1·26 per cent sodium bicarbonate for 0·9 per cent saline in the above regimen.

The diuresis is continued until the patient is fully conscious.

Forced Acid Diuresis

This regimen is indicated in severe acute amphetamine or quinine poisoning. It has also been advocated in severe fenfluramine poisoning.

Technique

1. Insert urinary catheter.
2. Intravenous infusion of:—

500 ml 5 per cent dextrose + 1·5 g
     ammonium chloride   }
500 ml 5 per cent dextrose   } in rotation.
500 ml 0·9 per cent saline   }

These fluids must be given at a rate of 1 litre in the first hour and 500 ml hourly thereafter. The regimen may have to be adjusted according to the patient's response and fluid and electrolyte balance.

The serum electrolytes *must* be measured hourly.

The urinary pH should be measured hourly and, if above 7·0, a further 1·5 g ammonium chloride should be added to the second bottle of 5 per cent dextrose in the above regimen. These patients often have marked hyperventilation and in these circumstances it may be very difficult to maintain an acid urine.

The diuresis is continued until the patient's condition is satisfactory.

Peritoneal Dialysis

Peritoneal dialysis, unlike haemodialysis, requires no elaborate equipment and little medical supervision. Once the catheter has been inserted in the peritoneum and the protocol for each exchange determined, further management can be regarded as a nursing procedure.

The evaluation of this procedure in a particular case demands a knowledge of the properties of the poison in question. This is somewhat difficult to acquire for a number of reasons. The peritoneal surface is not an inert colloid membrane, but a cellular structure possessing specialised properties of selective transudation, and so there are several characteristics of substances which influence their passage through this membrane. These include the molecular weight, the degree of ionisation of the substance and the extent and character of protein or lipid binding. The relative pH of the blood and of the dialysate, and the concentration gradient between the two will also influence the rate of the dialysability. For example, in acute phenobarbitone poisoning a blood level of 15 mg/100 ml is not uncommonly found and so there is a favourable gradient, whereas the toxic level of chlordiazepoxide (Librium) is in the region of 0·5 μg/100 ml providing a very poor and ineffective gradient.

The dialysate may be made hypertonic to increase the recovery of water soluble poison, or the pH, albumen or lipid content may be altered in order to encourage a particular poison in the blood to enter the dialysate. For example, in

acute phenobarbitone poisoning, if the dialysate is made
alkaline and albumen is added also, the recovery of active
drugs may be considerably increased. A further virtue of
peritoneal dialysis is that acid-base and electrolyte imbalance
may also be corrected by appropriate adjustments in the
constitution of the dialysing fluid.

The efficacy of peritoneal dialysis is considerably less than
that of haemodialysis and is probably about the same as
forced diuresis, although it is unwise to generalise[2, 7].

Unlike forced diuresis, there are very few contraindications
to peritoneal dialysis. Technical difficulty is likely to be
experienced from extensive peritoneal adhesions following
perforation of peptic ulceration or abdominal surgery.

Procedure

Pre-sterilised packs are now commercially available. This
pack supplies a specially designed trochar and cannula to
which must be attached a system of tubing to permit filling
of the peritoneal cavity and subsequent drainage by closed
gravitational drainage. There are also commercially prepared
solutions of fluids for peritoneal dialysis (Impersol).

For routine dialysis the standard 2 litre solution used for
each exchange is made up by adding:—

(a) Potassium chloride, 3 ml (5 ml contain 1 g KCl).

(b) Heparin, 1,000 units.

(c) Procaine, 1 per cent (2 ml).

If the patient is overhydrated this may be corrected by
adding to the above exchange fluid, glucose 50 per cent
(50 ml).

After bladder catheterisation, the dialysis catheter is inserted
in the midline of the abdomen three fingers breadth below
the umbilicus. The warmed dialysing fluid is then allowed to
flow by gravity from the reservoir into the peritoneum as
rapidly as possible. Usually less than 10 minutes are required
to run in the 2 litres used in an adult for each exchange. In
children or babies, the amount may be no more than 200 ml.
The time during which the dialysing fluid is left in the peri-

TABLE IV

SUBSTANCES WITH PROPERTIES FOR WHICH DIURESIS AND DIALYSIS MAY BE EFFECTIVE

The substances shown have properties which probably permit their removal by forced diuresis or peritoneal or haemodialysis. In many instances sufficient experience has not yet been accumulated to offer other than the range 0 = not dialysable through to + + + = readily dialysable. It should be clearly understood that the rating of certain substances is on the basis of perhaps only one reported case, and even that not necessarily well documented. Table IV, therefore, is but a very rough guide in certain instances.

Substance	Forced diuresis	Peritoneal dialysis	Haemodialysis	Comments
ALCOHOL ETHYL ALCOHOL	+ +	+ +	+ + +	
ALCOHOL METHYL ALCOHOL	+ +	+ +	+ + +	Recovery in P.D. will be enhanced if alkali is added to dialysate.
AMITRIPTYLINE (TRYPTIZOL)	0	0	0	
AMPHETAMINE	+ +	+ +	+ +	Forced diuresis with added ammonium chloride (p. 35) will increase elimination.
ANILINE	+ +	?	+ +	
BARBITURATES LONG ACTING	+ +	+ +	+ + +	See page 35 for forced diuresis. The recovery in P.D. will be increased by added albumen or THAM.
MEDIUM ACTING SHORT ACTING	0 0	+ +	+ +	
BORIC ACID	0	+ + +	+ + +	Do not attempt forced diuresis in view of possible renal failure.
BROMIDE	+ + +	+ + +	+ + +	
CARBON TETRACHLORIDE	0	+ +	+ +	Do not attempt forced diuresis in view of probable renal failure.
CHLORAL HYDRATE	+ + +	+ + +	+ + +	
CHLORDIAZEPOXIDE (LIBRIUM)	0	0	0	
CYCLOSERINE	+ +	+ + +	?	
DESIPRAMINE (PERTOFRAN)	0	0	0	

Substance	Forced diuresis	Peritoneal dialysis	Haemodialysis	Comments
DIAZEPAM (VALIUM)	0	0	0	
DICHLORALPHENAZINE (WELLDORM)	+++	+++	+++	
DIGITALIS	+	0	0	Mannitol diuresis only to be used. Haemodialysis may be dangerous.
ETHCHLORVYNOL (ARVYNOL)	0	+	+++	
ETHINAMATE (VALMIDATE)	?	0	++	
ETHYLENE GLYCOL	++	++	++	
FENFLURAMINE	++	++	++	Forced diuresis with added ammonium chloride (p. 35) will increase elimination.
FLUORIDE	+	?	+++	
GLUTETHIMIDE (DORIDEN)	0	+	+	Recovery may be increased by adding fat emulsion to the dialysate.
IMIPRAMINE (TOFRANIL)	0	0	0	
ISONIAZID	0	+	++	
LEAD	0	+	++	Dialysis should only be used in combination with chelating agents.
LITHIUM	+++	+++	+++	
MEPROBAMATE (EQUANIL)	++	0	+	
METHAQUALONE (QUAALUDE)	0	?	+	Forced diuresis should NOT be used in view of danger of pulmonary oedema.
METHAQUALONE + DIPHENHYDRAMINE (MANDRAX)	0	?	++	Haemodialysis is only appropriate if the blood level is above 12 mg. per cent in patients not tolerant to this drug. Forced diuresis should NOT be used in view of danger of pulmonary oedema.
METHYLPENTYNOL (OBLIVON)	+	+	+	
METHYPRYLONE (NOLUDAR)	+	+	+	
METHYL SALICYLATE	+++	+++	+++	Recovery will be increased by adding albumen to P.D. See page 34 for forced diuresis.

TABLE IV—*continued*

Substance	Forced diuresis	Peritoneal dialysis	Haemodialysis	Comments
MONOAMINE OXIDASE INHIBITORS	?	?	++	
MUSHROOM AMANITA PHALLOIDES	?	?	+++	Haemodialysis is unlikely to be effective more than 36 hours after ingestion.
MYSOLINE (PRIMIDONE)	++	++	+++	As for long acting barbiturate
NITRAZEPAM (MOGADON)	0	0	0	
NORTRIPTYLINE (AVENTYL)	0	0	0	
PARALDEHYDE	+	++	?	
PARACETAMOL	0	?	++	Haemodialysis is unlikely to be effective more than four hours after ingestion.
PENICILLIN	++	++	++	
PHENACETIN	0	?	++	Haemodialysis is unlikely to be effective more than four hours after ingestion.
PHENOTHIAZINES	0	0	0	
QUININE AND QUINIDINE	++	0	0	See page 35 for forced acid diuresis.
SALICYLATE	+++	+++	+++	Recovery will be increased by adding albumen to P.D. See page 34 for forced alkaline diuresis.
SODIUM CHLORATE	0	+++	+++	Do not attempt forced diuresis in view of probable renal failure.
STREPTOMYCIN	+	?	++	
SULPHONAMIDE	++	++	+++	
TRIMIPRAMINE (SURMONTIL)	0	0	0	

toneum may vary, but half an hour is the generally accepted optimum period. The fluid is then drained out by gravity and this usually takes 10 minutes; if the flow is sluggish the most likely fault is that the perforations on the cannula have become obstructed by bowel or omentum and slight repositioning of the cannula is usually all that is required.

The number of exchanges depends on the patient's condition but in general the dialysis should be continued until the patient is conscious. If the procedure is stopped at an earlier stage there is no means of assessing how much poison may still be present, for example in the bowel lumen or in the tissues. The dialysis may improve the patient's condition sufficiently for further mobilisation of the poison to occur and if the procedure has been stopped prematurely deterioration may occur.

Complications arising during and after the dialysis are few in contrast to dialysis for uraemia where infection is frequent; this complication is uncommon in patients treated for acute poisoning.

Haemodialysis

As with peritoneal dialysis an obvious but absolute requirement for this treatment to be effective is that the poison in its active form is dialysable. This procedure is the most efficient method but requires specialised technique and expert supervision and so is not described here.

Haemoperfusion—Ion Exchange Resins or Charcoal

Forced diuresis, peritoneal or haemodialysis and exchange transfusion all have marked limitations and to a lesser extent dangers in the treatment of severely poisoned patients. In view of this attempts have been made in recent years to develop alternative and safer methods of increasing elimination of toxic substances from the body.

In 1964 Edwards carried out *in vitro* tests for barbiturates using ion exchange resins. This method was used in 1971 by Rosenbaum in humans suffering from the same poisoning: largely because of technical difficulties this has not so far been generally accepted as a useful form of treatment.

Yatzidis in 1965 first employed a charcoal column to remove barbiturates from the blood of humans suffering from this poisoning. Dordoni in 1973 used the same methods to reduce plasma paracetamol. On occasions worth-while amounts of toxic substances can be removed by charcoal haemoperfusion, but hazards exist from charcoal embolisation with long term effects which are, as yet, unknown. Other dangers may arise from the charcoal removing important electrolytes, platelets and white blood cells. Strenuous efforts are being made to eliminate or reduce these hazards of ion exchange resins and charcoal haemoperfusion to an acceptable level. It is likely, therefore, that apparatus suitably modified will soon become available commercially. It is essential, however, that doctors keep these new forms of treatment in perspective and remember that the vast majority of patients with poisoning will recover very well with basic treatment alone and without aggressive methods of therapy to increase elimination of the poison.

REFERENCES

1 Maher, J. F. and Schreiner, G. E. (1968). *Trans. Amer. Soc. artif. intern Org.*, **14**, 440.

2 Bloomer, H. A. and Maddock, R. K. (1971). An assessment of diuresis and dialysis for treating acute barbiturate poisoning. In *Acute Barbiturate Poisoning*, ed. Matthew, H., p. 233. Excerpta Medica Monograph. Amsterdam: Excerpta Medica.

3 Mawer, G. E. and Lee, H. A. (1968). *Brit. med. J.*, **2**, 790.

4 Maddock, R. K. and Bloomer, H. A. (1968). *Clin. Res.*, **16**, 166.

5 Knochel, J. P., Clayton, L. E., Smith, W. L. and Barry, K. G. (1964). *J. Lab. clin. Med.*, **64**, 257.

6 Berlyne, G. M., Lee, H. A., Ralston, A. J. and Woodcock, J. A. (1966). *Lancet*, **2**, 75.

7 Hadden, J., Johnson, K., Smith, S., Price, L. and Giardina, E. (1969). *J. Am. med. Ass.*, **209**, 893.

8 Done, A. K. (1969). *Pharmacol. for Phycns.*, **3**, 1.

9 Yatzidis, H. (1971). The use of ion exchange resins and charcoal in acute barbiturate poisoning. In *Acute Barbiturate Poisoning*, ed. Matthew, H., p. 223. Excerpta Medica Monograph. Amsterdam: Excerpta Medica.

CHAPTER 7

BASIC PRINCIPLES OF PSYCHIATRIC TREATMENT

As already indicated, the incidence of acute poisoning has risen in a most dramatic and alarming way during the past 25 years. Accidental poisoning, particularly in children, has contributed considerably to this overall rise but the real increase in poisoning is due to what used to be called 'attempted suicide'. The vast majority of patients who have taken poison do not genuinely wish to die; it is clear that the motives leading up to their admission to hospital are very varied. In order to draw attention to this distinction it is helpful to use the term 'self-poisoning' to describe the act[1]. This is a far more general concept and does not indicate motive in itself. It is preferable to restrict the term 'attempted suicide' to those patients who appear to have a very determined desire to end their life.

The basic reason for a self-poisoning act may be regarded as a desire to produce a change in the environment, which to the particular individual in question, cannot be achieved by any more rational means[2]. These patients may express this desire in a variety of ways—'I was fed up', 'I couldn't go on any longer', 'I just wanted to sleep'. Their fundamental wish is for a flight into oblivion. Whilst such acts may be considered as essentially manipulative—and so perhaps engender antipathy towards the patient—it is important to remember that they may be an expression of severe distress or severe illness. In practice many patients with self-poisoning are found to be distressed but not necessarily ill. Often it becomes clear that, in fact, the one admitted may not be necessarily the member of the family most in need of help. The self-poisoning incident

43

is intended simply to draw attention to illness in another important family member. The impulsive qualities of the self-poisoning act may be very impressive. Alcohol is frequently taken and may precipitate such behaviour.

So common are self-poisoning incidents nowadays, that this behaviour has now taken the place of Victorian vapours and hysteria as a means of expressing distress, frustration, or merely rebellion. For example the type of situation in which this behaviour is frequently found is where quarrels arise between a boy friend and a girl friend or between husband and wife. Rather than settle the issue by logical and rational discussion, one or other partner takes an overdose of tablets in the hope that by so doing the partner will feel acute remorse. In practice, there is little doubt that this tactic is often successful. It is not uncommon to see relatives arriving in the ward extremely concerned and agitated, laden with chocolates and bunches of flowers, etc. Clearly a favourable outcome has been achieved at the expense of the remorse of the relatives, and all is forgiven. On occasions, however, tragedy may occur, and an act which was meant to be merely manipulative, may end in fatality.

At the present time, self-poisoning accounts for some 80 per cent of admissions to the Edinburgh Poisoning Treatment Centre. True attempted suicide is probably present in only 10 per cent of admissions and a further 10 per cent are considered genuinely accidental.

It is therefore most important to appreciate that management of the patient with acute poisoning is by no means completed with physical recovery. Psychiatric assessment is essential in all patients even where it may seem that the circumstances are those of accidental poisoning. It is a common mistake for doctors to give their patients the 'benefit of the doubt' in this regard, with possibly tragic consequences. A common problem of this type is when an elderly person who resides alone is admitted suffering from coal gas poisoning. On account of frailty, partial blindness and tendency to confusion such an episode is often regarded as accidental, whereas it is really an act of self-poisoning committed by a depressed, lonely person.

In the past, the severity of the physical illness resulting from the self-administered poisoning, was often held to be a measure of the degree of the underlying psychiatric illness. In practice this is by no means true, for there are many very disturbed people who by virtue of extreme mental agitation become so disorganised that they take quite small quantities of poison and come to little harm. Others have doubts after starting to take a large quantity of tablets, whilst many people take only what they consider to be 'enough'. Fortunately the toxicity of the drugs is frequently overestimated. From the point of view of adequate psychiatric management, it is vital to remember that the size of the overdose may in no way parallel the severity of the underlying psychological or sociological upset[3].

Acute poisoning, and more particularly acute self-poisoning, is therefore a crisis situation and should be regarded as such and not minimised or dismissed. The role of the psychiatrist is clear. He must obtain as quickly as possible a comprehensive picture of the events related to the self-poisoning incident. With this in view, he should interview the patient as soon as the mental and physical state permits. It is most important to interview patients and relatives before the facts leading to the poisoning act become obscured or perhaps rationalised, and thereby important factors might be withheld. The psychiatric social worker must also be involved and interview the nearest relatives or the most important family member as soon as possible[4]. Further information may have to be obtained from other relatives, friends or work associates or from hospital or social agencies. As a result of the information gained, it should be possible to decide which member of the family unit requires further investigation or possibly treatment. The crisis situation often provides an excellent opportunity for the patient to accept psychiatric care.

The figures obtained for psychiatric illness in the Edinburgh Poisons Unit are shown in Table V. The patients in the

TABLE V

PSYCHIATRIC ILLNESS IN POISONED PATIENTS

Depressive illness	25 per cent
Personality disorder	25 per cent
Alcoholic problems and/or drug addiction . .	21 per cent
No definite psychiatric disorder	29 per cent

group who were regarded as having no psychiatric illness
had previously shown adjustment which seemed satisfactory
and the actual incident of self-poisoning could be related to
some very recent stress.   As many patients in each group
took their overdose after drinking alcohol this obviously
played a considerable part.   The psychiatric disposal of these
patients is shown in Table VI.   Less than half of the patients

TABLE VI

PSYCHIATRIC REQUIREMENTS ON DISCHARGE

Transferred to psychiatric in-patient treatment . .	25 per cent
Only psychiatric out-patient treatment required .	23 per cent
Psychiatric social worker to continue supervision .	25 per cent
No further psychiatric follow-up required . .	27 per cent

were treated subsequently in psychiatric hospitals or as
psychiatric out-patients.   Of the remainder obviously some
refused help and others were thought unsuitable for treatment,
but this left a large group of people, some of whom continued
to need social help and support or even supervision in the
community.   This support must be supplied by social agencies
and much of the burden in this situation falls on the psychiatric
social worker, mental health officer or health visitor.   In many
other people the self-poisoning episodes temporarily or
permanently ease the crisis and no further immediate help
may be required.   However, these individuals are often still
'at risk' by virtue of some degree of personality abnormality
or because of tenuous levels of adaptation.   Particularly vulner-
able in this respect are adolescent girls and young married
women.   An important aspect of management, therefore, is to

attempt to anticipate the crisis in such groups, and if necessary, seek the help of the psychiatrist. Distressing insomnia may occur for about 10 days after recovery of consciousness. It is important to recognise this upset which responds best to administration of chlorpromazine. A recent study[5] has demonstrated the importance of detailed hospital assessment in the prevention of repeated acts of self-poisoning.

A common cause of a false sense of security is the misconception that persons who voice thoughts of suicide will not, in fact, commit the act. This is far from true and their reference to suicide should always be taken seriously.

In summary, therefore, good medicine demands the recognition and treatment of the patient's plea for help which is expressed as self-poisoning.

REFERENCES

1 Kessel, N. (1965). *Brit. med. J.*, **2**, 1265 and 1336.
2 Kessel, N. (1971). Psychiatric aspects of acute barbiturate poisoning. in *Acute Barbiturate Poisoning*, ed. Matthew, H., p. 269. Excerpta Medica Monograph. Amsterdam: Excerpta Medica.
3 Matthew, H., Proudfoot, A. T., Brown, S. S. and Aitken, R. C. B. (1969). *Brit. med. J.*, **3**, 489.
4 McCulloch, J. W. (1971). Social aspects of acute barbiturate poisoning. In *Acute Barbiturate Poisoning*, ed. Matthew, H., p. 291. Excerpta Medica Monograph. Amsterdam: Excerpta Medica.
5 Kennedy, P. (1972). *Brit. med. J.*, **4**, 255.

CHAPTER 8

ACUTE BARBITURATE POISONING

Despite authoritative advice that barbiturates have no place in therapy except as anticonvulsants, doctors in Britain continue to prescribe vast amounts. Prescriptions for barbiturates number 14 million per annum for a population of 55 million, the average amount in each prescription being 60 tablets or capsules. Over the past five years, however, it is encouraging that decreasing amounts have been prescribed. Nevertheless, acute barbiturate poisoning accounts for about 70 per cent of the total mortality due to acute ingestant poisoning[1]: in Britain there are 2,000 adult deaths from this cause each year[2]. In addition, barbiturates are in most countries still the commonest drug involved in self-poisoning[3] and are the drug most frequently chosen by those taking drugs for 'kicks'[4]. Acute barbiturate poisoning, therefore, remains a common condition, which every doctor will encounter during the course of his professional life.

Traditionally it is the practice to divide the barbiturate drugs into long acting, medium acting, short acting and ultra short acting classes (Table VII). The duration of the hypnotic action of these types depends largely on their rate of absorption from the alimentary tracts, the degree of lipid solubility and to a lesser extent on the degree of protein binding. In therapeutic dosage, there is no doubt that this classification is not only a useful, but also an accurate measure of the action of these drugs. In acute overdosage, however, shortness of action should not be equated with lack of toxicity. It is a common error to feel reassured when the patient is known to have taken a 'short acting barbiturate', the interpretation being that the patient will only remain unconscious for a

TABLE VII

CLASSIFICATION OF BARBITURATES

	Duration of Action in therapeutic dose	Official name	Proprietary name
Long Acting	{12–24 hours 8–16 hours 12–24 hours	Barbitone Sodium barbitone Phenobarbitone	Veronal Medinal Luminal
Medium Acting	8–10 hours 8–10 hours 8–10 hours	Allobarbitone Butobarbitone Amylobarbitone	Dial Soneryl Amytal
Short Acting	6–8 hours 4–6 hours 4–6 hours	Pentobarbitone Cyclobarbitone Quinalbarbitone	Nembutal Phanodorm Seconal
Ultra-short Acting	{3–4 hours 3–4 hours	Hexobarbitone Thiopentone	Evipan Pentothal

relatively short period of time. This is fallacious. In fact, although it is true to say that patients who have taken, for example, an overdose of phenobarbitone may remain unconscious for a prolonged period of time, they tend to remain at a somewhat safer level of unconsciousness than patients who have taken a large overdose of, for example, quinalbarbitone (Seconal). Moreover ill-effects from overdosage, such as severe shock or respiratory failure are more frequent and more serious with medium and short acting barbiturates. In addition, it will be seen that the active therapy available for these different groups of barbiturates is more restricted with medium and short-acting drugs than it is with the long acting. Overdosage therefore with the former types of barbiturate should be regarded with the graver concern.

The number of proprietary preparations of barbiturates is extremely great. The picture is even more complicated by virtue of the fact that many of them, for example Tuinal contain both a short acting barbiturate, quinalbarbitone, and a medium acting, amylobarbitone, whilst other proprietary preparations, such as Drinamyl, contain both a barbiturate and an unrelated drug, dexamphetamine sulphate, which is a central nervous system stimulant.

Assessment of Severity of Poisoning

It is frequently suggested that measurements of blood levels provide a satisfactory means of assessing how severely a patient is poisoned by barbiturate drugs[5]. This supposition is fallacious, both because of the individual variation in the rate of metabolism of the barbiturate and in tissue tolerance (p. 16). A further fallacy was introduced by the difficulty of devising a standard method of chemical assay. A commonly used method of assay is that of Broughton[6]. In urine this method measures non-toxic barbiturate metabolites as well as the active drug, and therefore the estimated result may give a misleadingly high impression of the active drug present. Secondly, methods of extraction of the barbiturate from test samples prior to measurement by the Broughton method of assay vary, and therefore different series of blood or urine levels may not necessarily be comparable. Thirdly, if a number of other drugs have been taken there will be interference with the measurement of barbiturate. Although, in recent years, these problems may be overcome by the use of gas liquid chromatography, it cannot be too strongly stressed that the assessment must depend on the clinical features present, and in particular, on the impairment of level of consciousness and the presence or absence of findings such as respiratory failure, 'shock' and hypothermia.

Clinical Features of Overdosage

CENTRAL NERVOUS SYSTEM. Barbiturates act on the central nervous system as depressants. The primary clinical features are therefore those of impaired level of consciousness. Accurate assessment of this level is, in practice, the most satisfactory means of assessing the severity of the poisoning itself. It must be understood, however, that serious complications may occur when the patient is not deeply unconscious and these require consideration in a full assessment. The Reed classification of severity of poisoning[7] attempts to allow for these, but in our experience provides no practical advantages over our simpler concept. The system of grading of levels of consciousness indicated (p. 18) provides a useful objective means of comparing the relative severity of overdosage in different patients. As stated, the standard painful stimulus is rubbing of the clenched fist on the patient's sternum. This method of assessing response has clear advantages over other means that have been recommended. Thus supra-orbital pressure with the finger should be avoided as there is a danger of the finger slipping, with possible damage to the eye of the patient. The state of the pupils is considered by many to be a good index of the level of severity of the poisoning but in practice the pupils may be quite normal or very small and show poor response to light, or they may be very widely dilated. These findings are so variable and so inconsistent that they provide little or no index of the condition of the patient. Similarly, the peri-

pheral limb reflexes may be extremely variable. Withdrawal
features occur mainly in patients habituated to barbiturates,
but these may happen even when the individual has taken
the drug for a comparatively short time. The main features
are restlessness, insomnia, delirium, hallucinations and
convulsions. The hallucinations are usually visual.

RESPIRATORY SYSTEM. The effects on respiration are the
most life-threatening and result from the direct depressant
action upon the respiratory centre. This leads not only to a
reduction in the respiratory rate, but frequently also to hypo-
ventilation. In addition to clinical observation of cyanosis
and shallow respiration, a useful means of assessing respiratory
failure in this type of poisoning is provided by a Wright's
spirometer. If there is any doubt regarding the efficacy of
respiratory function, arterial blood gas studies should be
made (p. 20).

CARDIOVASCULAR SYSTEM. Barbiturate drugs have two
major effects upon the cardiovascular system. There is a direct
toxic effect on the myocardium, and the tone of the muscu-
lature of the peripheral vessels may also be reduced resulting
in excessive capillary exudation and venous pooling in the
lower limbs both of which contribute to an effective hypovolaemia and subsequent diminution in the venous return to
the heart. Finally, in the most severe cases of poisoning
central nervous system depression may be of such a degree
that the cardiovascular centre becomes involved.

HYPOTHERMIA. Significant hypothermia (p. 27) is frequently
found in patients with acute barbiturate poisoning, and
occasionally it may be so severe as to require specific therapy.
During recovery it is important to appreciate that pyrexia
will almost invariably occur. Return to normality occurs
spontaneously after a period of some hours or possibly days.
This fever does not necessarily mean the presence of infection
and should not be viewed with undue concern.

GASTROINTESTINAL SYSTEM. A useful means of assessing the severity of poisoning is to relate the presence or absence of bowel sounds to the overall condition of the patient. For example, unconsciousness with the absence of bowel sounds usually indicates that the patient is severely poisoned, and that it is unlikely that he is absorbing any more of the drug at that particular time. During the period of recovery, bowel sounds may be heard at a reasonably early stage, but the return of bowel function should be viewed with considerable caution since, if there is more drug in the bowel lumen, further absorption may occur. As a result, it is not at all uncommon for the level of consciousness to fluctuate during the period of recovery of a deeply unconscious patient. Conversely, if when an unconscious patient is first seen bowel sounds are present this may indicate that he will become more deeply unconscious should there be drug still left in the bowel to be absorbed. In short, patients who are unconscious and lack bowel sounds may be regarded as being severely poisoned; those who have bowel sounds present may be less severely ill but should nevertheless be observed closely in the anticipation of possible worsening.

RENAL SYSTEM. Impairment of renal function is likely to develop when there is severe hypotension, but it is more commonly seen in patients who are significantly hypothermic. With correct management renal failure rarely occurs but on occasion it may result from the over-enthusiastic use of vasopressor drugs in the treatment of hypotension[8]. This danger cannot be over-stressed and the precautions described (p. 21) must be observed with great care if this complication is to be avoided.

DERMATOLOGICAL SYSTEM. A feature of acute barbiturate poisoning is the development of bullous lesions (p. 12) which occur in 6 per cent of patients with this condition. These develop at an early stage and provide a good clinical indication of this poisoning[9, 10].

Treatment

The principles of intensive supportive therapy (p. 18) must form the basis of management of acute barbiturate poisoning. Provided the regimen is applied with sufficient vigour and attention to detail, and that the use of analeptic drugs is avoided, at least 95 per cent of all patients presenting with acute barbiturate intoxication will be treated successfully by this management alone. The therapy has been proved to be entirely suitable even for many severely poisoned patients.

It is, of course, a logical approach to the treatment of any poisoning to try to remove it from the body. In recent years the use of methods such as forced osmotic alkaline diuresis and haemodialysis to increase the elimination of the drug have been advocated even for patients who are apparently only mildly poisoned. Others have suggested that by using these special methods the period of unconsciousness may be reduced to as little as one-third of that achieved by intensive supportive therapy[11]. Such studies, however, have used a comparison with control groups of patients which is by no means satisfactory because of the very wide individual variation in response to these drugs. At the present time there is no satisfactory means of assessing how long any individual patient will remain unconscious.

With few exceptions, the reports describing these methods of treatment indicate that only the equivalent of one or two capsules of the drug may be recovered even when the overdosage taken has been large. Whilst a genuine recovery of several grams of barbiturate would justify this form of treatment, it has already been mentioned that quantitative estimation of barbiturate depends on the method of extraction of the drug from the test sample prior to measurement. In considering reports of high recoveries, therefore, it must be borne in mind that non-toxic, water soluble metabolites of the drug may be included in the quantitation, and that the recovery of the active principle may be low[12]. Even with haemodialysis, which is the most efficient method of removing dialysable poisons, only small quantities of the active drug are removed, except in barbitone and phenobarbitone poisoning[13]. On the basis of clinical impression, it has been suggested that the removal of even small amounts may be of considerable pharmacological and clinical significance. There is at the present time, however, no objective evidence to substantiate this claim. A further objection to the use of these special methods of removal of the poison is that none of them are without risk in themselves, and it would therefore appear inappropriate to introduce another possible hazard to the patient when simpler and more suitable methods of treatment are available.

In summary it must be emphasised that the assessment of the patient must be a clinical assessment. In the great majority of patients the regimen of intensive supportive therapy is adequate. Special methods to remove the poison should only be used in severely ill patients in whom intensive supportive therapy fails to prevent deterioration. There is moreover considerable doubt as to whether these methods will be therapeutically effective except in patients suffering from barbitone or phenobarbitone intoxication.

REFERENCES

1 Barraclough, B. M., Nelson, B., Bunch, J. and Sainsbury, P. (1971). *J. Roy. Coll. Gen. Practit.*, **21**, 645.
2 Barraclough, B. M. (1974). *Lancet*, **1**, 57.
3 Matthew, H. (1972-3). *Prevent*, **1**, 57.
4 Forrest, J. A. H. and Tarala, R. A. (1973). *Brit. med. J.*, **4**, 136.
5 Lawson, A. A. H. and Proudfoot, A. T. (1971). In *Acute Barbiturate Poisoning*, ed. Matthew, H., p. 179. Amsterdam: Excerpta Medica.
6 Broughton, P. M. G. (1956). *Biochem. J.*, **63**, 207.
7 Reed, C. E., Driggs, M. F. and Foote, C. C. (1952). *Ann. Intern. Med.*, **37**, 290.
8 Shubin, H. and Weil, M. H. (1965). *Amer. J. Med.*, **38**, 853.
9 Beveridge, G. W. and Lawson, A. A. H. (1965). *Brit. med. J.*, **1**, 835.
10 Beveridge, G. W. (1971). *Brit. med. J.*, **4**, 116.
11 Myschetzky, A. and Lassen, N. A. (1963). *J. Amer. Med. Ass.*, **185**, 936.
12 Bloomer, H. A. and Maddock, R. K. (1971). In *Acute Barbiturate Poisoning*, ed. Matthew, H., p. 233. Amsterdam: Excerpta Medica.
13 Setter, J. G., Maher, J. F. and Schreiner, G. E. (1966). *Arch. Int. Med.*, **117**, 224.

CHAPTER 9

POISONING BY TOXIC INHALANTS

There are many poisonous substances, gases and vapours which may be absorbed readily following inhalation. A number of these are very toxic and may result in severe acute poisoning after a short period of exposure. As some of these poisons are used commonly in industry and as pesticides, accidental poisoning is not uncommon, but they may also feature in self-poisoning and even genuine suicidal incidents.

Some of the poisonings described in this chapter may occur by means other than inhalation, but these are included for convenience.

Acute Carbon Monoxide Poisoning

Acute poisoning due to the inhalation of air or fumes containing carbon monoxide remains the commonest cause of death of all acute poisonings in adults. These deaths, however, occur predominantly shortly after exposure and at the scene of the poisoning. Although it is in itself a very dangerous form of poisoning, the major factor in the mortality is that it is most frequently encountered in elderly patients who often have serious underlying pathological disorders of the cardio-vascular, respiratory and central nervous systems. As a result of this, the effects of the poisoning, which are mainly due to hypoxia, become more apparent.

The major source of carbon monoxide is town gas but it is found in significant quantities wherever incomplete combustion occurs, and particularly in the exhaust fumes from motor vehicles. It is therefore a common toxic agent and the risks of exposure to it are considerable. In many parts of Britain the content of carbon monoxide in household gas has been reduced from 25 per cent to 5 per cent. It should be noted, however, that this remains a dangerous concentration. Also in more recent years many household gas supplies have been converted from coal gas to natural gas, which is not in itself toxic except in very high concentration, when it may cause asphyxiation. Carbon monoxide poisoning may still occur, however, when inappropriate appliances are used due to the incomplete combustion of natural gas.

Carbon monoxide in itself is a colourless, odourless gas with an affinity for haemoglobin 300 times that of oxygen[1]; as a result of the conversion of haemoglobin to carboxyhaemo-globin the oxygen-carrying power of the arterial blood is diminished and hypoxia results. There is also evidence that carbon monoxide may have a direct toxic effect on the myocardium[2].

Pathological Effects

There is considerable discussion regarding the sequence of events leading to the damage to major functions which occurs in this poisoning. Carbon monoxide poisoning may be regarded as occurring in two distinct phases. There is an initial hypoxic period which ceases very soon after the patient is removed from the poisonous atmosphere. Secondly, however, and often of more clinical importance, is the vicious circle which develops from the primary hypoxia. Capillary damage occurs with resultant tissue oedema in general and of the cerebral tissue in particular; local hypoxia thus intervenes and leads to further capillary damage. The second phase may well persist even when carboxyhaemoglobin in the circulating blood has been reduced to low or even negligible levels. Irreversible brain damage may occur as a result of either primary or secondary hypoxia[3, 4]. It is important to recognise that in either case with appropriate measures to reduce the oedema, and particularly cerebral oedema, it is frequently possible to prevent the onset of irreversible neurological damage. Such damage precedes failure of breathing and circulation. When a patient is first seen there is no means of telling how close he is to final collapse, since when the latter two functions fail they do so within a period of a few minutes of each other. During this brief interval of time the patient is in an extremely critical condition. Survival very much depends on how quickly adequate therapy is given. It must be stressed therefore that all patients with this poisoning should be regarded as being in a critical condition and appropriate resuscitatory measures must be put in hand immediately.

Clinical Features

When carbon monoxide poisoning is due to exposure to town gas the characteristic smell of the patient's breath and clothing usually makes the diagnosis clear. Since major toxic effects of the poisoning result from either primary or secondary hypoxia, the severity depends on the character of the original blood supply. Elderly patients therefore, with extensive atheroma are much more 'at risk' than young patients with perfectly healthy circulations. Similarly, pre-existing pathology due to myocardial infarction, cerebrovascular accident, chronic lung disease or similar conditions, has a particularly significant influence on the prognosis. All these factors can contribute to the severity of the hypoxia.

CENTRAL NERVOUS SYSTEM. The effects on the central nervous system range from acute agitation and mental confusion to deep coma. Features of agitation frequently occur when cerebral oedema is present, and therefore they are often associated with papilloedema, hypertonia, increase in peripheral limb reflexes, and possibly extensor plantar responses. Patients who are very agitated are commonly found to have marked negativism and lack of co-operation, which may closely resemble acute hysteria. It is important to recognise this apparent hysteria as evidence of severe poisoning, which may be a prelude to deepening coma and irreversible brain damage. Hyperpyrexia may be considerable.

The sequelae of damage to the central nervous system may be tragic and include monoplegia or hemiplegia. Impairment of higher intellectual function, personality changes, cerebellar damage and severe Parkinsonism all may occur and may be delayed by several weeks after apparent initial recovery. Localised or extensive cerebral atrophy may occur. An uncommon consequence of coal gas poisoning when there is marked damage to the mid-brain and basal ganglia is akinetic mutism.

CARDIOVASCULAR SYSTEM. The incidence of myocardial damage, as shown by electrocardiography is much more frequent than would be suspected on clinical grounds. Damage to the myocardium may result in tachycardia, various arrhythmias, hypotension and shock. Acute myocardial infarction may develop. Myocardial ischaemia, but not necessarily actual infarction, is almost invariable in severe carbon monoxide poisonings at all ages[5].

RESPIRATORY SYSTEM. In severe poisonings the marked degree of hypoxia initially provides a powerful stimulus to the respiratory centre and the patient therefore, may have rapid respiration. Acute congestion and oedema of the lungs may occur and respiratory failure may follow, and is usually a terminal feature[3]. Pulmonary atelectasis as a result of inhalation of vomit may occur, particularly in patients in whom the level of consciousness is impaired.

GASTROINTESTINAL SYSTEM. Patients with moderate or severe carbon monoxide poisoning frequently have marked nausea, and vomiting, and incontinence of faeces is common. Haematemesis and melaena may also occur.

EFFECTS ON SKIN. The pink colour, due to carboxyhaemoglobin, of the mucous membranes and of the skin which is described in so many textbooks of forensic medicine is very uncommon in clinical practice, but when present indicates a severe degree of poisoning. The colour is fairly characteristic of carbon monoxide intoxication but its absence by no means excludes this diagnosis. Skin pallor is a much more frequent finding. Bullous eruptions may occur in carbon monoxide poisoning[6]. These tend to be discrete and isolated lesions.

E

The bullous fluid is usually thick and cellular and there is often an inflammatory reaction in the surrounding skin. These bullae are almost certainly localised by external pressure, but the factor predisposing to the formation of blisters is skin hypoxia. They occur less frequently than in acute barbiturate poisoning (p. 53) and seldom involve the fingers and toes. Cold perspiration may be a striking feature.

Treatment

This must be begun as a matter of great urgency.
1. The patient must be removed from exposure to the poisonous atmosphere.
2. The principles of intensive supportive therapy (p. 18) apply equally to poisoning due to carbon monoxide, as to any ingestant. In particular, care of the respiratory tract is of great importance. There is considerable controversy as to whether one should give 100 per cent oxygen or a mixture of 95 per cent oxygen and 5 per cent carbon dioxide using a mechanical system which prevents rebreathing. It would seem logical that in a condition in which a patient is suffering from marked hypoxia 100 per cent oxygen would be the more suitable. In patients who have ceased to breathe spontaneously there is such an accumulation of endogenous carbon dioxide that to give more exogenous carbon dioxide is unreasonable. For these patients 100 per cent oxygen should be given together with assisted respiration. Even when the patient is breathing spontaneously, however, the respiratory centre may still be depressed by hypoxia resulting from a high carboxyhaemoglobin level. In these circumstances removal of the carbon monoxide from the circulating blood is an urgent matter and the respiratory stimulant effect of the mixture of 95 per cent oxygen and 5 per cent carbon dioxide is a valuable addition to the treatment[7].
3. In patients showing any evidence, or even suspicion, of cerebral oedema rapid reduction of the oedema is a matter of urgency. Intravenous infusion of 500 ml of 20 per cent

mannitol should be given over 15 minutes followed by 500 ml of 5 per cent dextrose over the next four hours.

4. In view of the high incidence of myocardial ischaemia and indeed infarction, the patient should be kept at rest for a period of three days while the degree of possible damage is being assessed.

Hyperbaric Oxygen

There is no doubt that the elimination of carbon monoxide from the blood is increased markedly by the use of oxygen under pressure. In addition, at two atmospheres pressure, the oxygen carried as oxyhaemoglobin increases by 1 volume per cent, whereas the amount carried in physical solution in the plasma increases from 0·25 volumes to 3·8 volumes per cent, which greatly increases the diffusion from plasma to cells. Therefore, hyperbaric oxygen has a beneficial effect on both phases of carbon monoxide poisoning. There are, however, disadvantages to hyperbaric oxygen and these may be considered under two headings.

Theoretical Objections

Few studies have been done on humans. Much of the work on the use of hyperbaric oxygen in the treatment of carbon monoxide poisoning has been done in animals[7], most showing an initial carboxyhaemoglobin level of approximately 70 per cent. It is very uncommon however, for patients admitted to hospital to have blood levels as high as this, and even those deeply unconscious may have levels of barely 40 per cent. It is known that a human can withstand a loss of 40 per cent of the oxygen carrying power of the blood without any ill-effects provided the initial haemoglobin level is normal. It seems unlikely, therefore, that the use of the hyperbaric chamber in hospital would save very many patients from the lethal effects of primary anoxia. Moreover, the use of hyperbaric oxygen has been shown to increase the cerebrovascular resistance by 55 per cent with a resultant 25 per cent decrease in cerebral blood flow.

Practical Objections

Most chambers take approximately 20 minutes to reach full working pressure. Reference to disocciation curves for carboxyhaemoglobin shows that in gassed animals blood carboxyhaemoglobin falls below a danger level in approximately 20 minutes. To this 20 minutes delay should be added the further period of time elapsing between the patient being found and subsequently admitted to hospital, which in practice, usually takes longer than one hour. It is most unlikely therefore, that the use of hyperbaric oxygen treatment will be effective in the primary anoxic phase. Secondary hypoxia, on the other hand, may benefit from the increased oxygen diffusion gradient produced by hyperbaric oxygen and where available it has a place in treatment. Cerebral oedema however is almost always relieved by simpler measures, such as the infusion of hypertonic mannitol or glucose.

The major objection is therefore of a practical nature and it would seem that this method of treatment, which is expensive both in equipment and in staffing, is not vital in the management of these patients. In some areas portable hyperbaric chambers to be taken to the scene of the gassing are available. The value of this advance in treatment remains to be fully assessed but as yet there is no convincing evidence that the use of hyperbaric oxygen offers any real advantages.

Kerosene and Other Petroleum Distillates[1, 2]

Although seldom seen in Great Britain, kerosene poisoning is common in children in other countries. In the United States, for example, approximately 30,000 poisonings occur in children under the age of five each year. This is not surprising as kerosene and petroleum distillates are constituents of many domestic cleaning fluids, furniture polishes and paint thinners (turpentine substitute), quite apart from common use as illuminating and heating fuels. Kerosene is irritant to the gastrointestinal tract and, if absorbed depresses the central nervous system. Aspiration into the lungs is a particular danger. On account of its low surface tension and high vapour pressure even a few millilitres of kerosene entering the respiratory passages will spread throughout the lungs resulting in severe pneumonitis. Kerosene is not readily absorbed after ingestion.

Clinical Features

Mild poisoning following inhalation causes symptoms resembling alcoholic inebriation. More severe poisoning produces the following features:—

GASTROINTESTINAL SYSTEM. Nausea, vomiting, diarrhoea.

RESPIRATORY SYSTEM. If inhaled or aspirated, intense pulmonary congestion and chemical pneumonitis.

CENTRAL NERVOUS SYSTEM. Headache, blurring of vision, vertigo and tinnitus. Restlessness, excitement, inco-ordination, disorientation, delirium which may deteriorate into coma and convulsions.

Respiratory failure is the usual mode of death.

Treatment

1. It is vital to prevent aspiration into the lungs. Therefore *do not* attempt emesis or gastric aspiration and lavage in a conscious or semi-conscious patient. The one exception to this is when the patient is sufficiently unconscious to allow endotracheal intubation following which gastric aspiration and lavage may be performed.
2. Absorption of ingested kerosene can be slowed by giving 250 ml of liquid paraffin orally.
3. If there is suspicion of chemical pneumonitis hydrocortisone (100 mg) intramuscularly at six-hourly intervals for 48 hours together with benzylpenicillin in full dosage for seven days should be given.
4. Respiratory depression may need appropriate treatment (p. 19) and convulsions should be treated with intravenous diazepam or intramuscular sodium phenobarbitone.

Carbon Tetrachloride

This compound is widely used as a solvent for removing grease both in the home and in industry, and in medicine for removing adhesive plaster and as an anthelmintic. It has been used in some types of fire extinguishers but because it decomposes to phosgene on heating it is now being replaced for this purpose by other polyhalogenated hydrocarbons. Carbon tetrachloride is very toxic to all types of cells, but especially to those of the liver and kidney[1, 2]. If taken with alcohol, absorption is considerably increased. It may also be absorbed by 'sniffing for kicks'. The fatal dose for an adult by inhalation or ingestion can be as low as 3 ml.

Clinical Features

The signs and symptoms of acute toxicity are similar whether following inhalation or ingestion, but following the latter the gastrointestinal upset is more marked.

ALIMENTARY SYSTEM. Sore throat, nausea, vomiting, severe abdominal colic.

CENTRAL NERVOUS SYSTEM. Headache, dizziness; stupor and convulsions may occur, leading to loss of consciousness.

CARDIOVASCULAR SYSTEM. Bradycardia with hypotension is usually present but there is also a tendency to serious ventricular arrhythmias.

RESPIRATORY SYSTEM. Respiratory depression.

HEPATIC AND RENAL DISORDERS. If the patient survives the acute phase then after two to three days features of hepatic and renal damage may appear. In very severe poisoning, however, these features may occur in the first 12 hours.

Treatment

1. Remove contaminated clothing.
2. Gastric aspiration and lavage (p. 23) if the poison has been ingested.
3. Intensive supportive therapy (p 18).
4. Treatment of acute renal and hepatic failure may be required.

Cyanide

Although poisoning by hydrogen cyanide is uncommon this substance and its salts are extensively used in the chemical industry. They are very toxic but antidotes are available. Cyanide poisoning may arise from the inhalation of hydrocyanic acid vapour and by percutaneous absorption, as well as by ingestion. Cyanide inhibits cytochrome B, one of the enzymes necessary for oxygen transport at cellular level. It is one of the most rapidly acting poisons and death from asphyxia may occur within a few minutes, but may be delayed for a number of hours. Agents which bind cyanide more strongly than the iron of cytochrome can reverse the inhibition. This principle is utilised in the specific therapy for cyanide poisoning[1, 2].

The administration of nitrite induces methaemoglobinaemia. Cyanmethaemoglobin is then formed preferentially and is relatively non-toxic. Sodium thiosulphate is then injected to provide adequate amounts of substrate to detoxify the cyanide of the cyanmethaemoglobin by converting it to thiocyanate[3].

Clinical Features

The speed of onset of symptoms and signs will obviously depend on the quantity of cyanide absorbed. With a low concentration in air or when swallowed in small amounts on a full stomach, headache, dyspnoea, vomiting, ataxia and loss of consciousness occur gradually. If a large amount is absorbed the features appear very rapidly, and the patient becomes deeply unconscious. The smell of bitter almonds is not necessarily present. The skin remains pink unless breathing has ceased even though respiration is markedly depressed. The pulse is rapid and of poor volume and the heart sounds very feeble. The blood pressure may not be recordable. The limb reflexes are absent and the pupils dilated. The patient may continue in this state even for hours, but as long as the heart sounds are audible there are good grounds for expecting recovery.

Treatment

Speed is absolutely essential. There is debate about the relative merits of chelation as opposed to detoxication by nitrites. We recommend the chelating agent cobalt edetate available commercially as Kelocyanor[4, 5]. An initial 40 ml intravenous injection of 600 mg is given over one minute. This may cause hypotension, tachycardia and sometimes retching. Recovery is likely within a further minute, but if this does not occur, an injection of 300 mg should be given immediately. This should be followed by 50 ml 5 per cent dextrose intravenously.

Specially prepared kits for the alternative nitrite treatment are available but the chemicals contained may deteriorate.

1. If the poisoning is due to inhalation, remove from contaminated atmosphere.

2. Break an ampoule of amyl nitrite under the patient's nose, forcing the vapour into the lungs. One ampoule should be inhaled for 10 second periods at three minute intervals. During this procedure inject 10 ml 3 per cent sodium nitrite intravenously over three minutes.

3. Artificial respiration with oxygen should then be administered[6].

4. Inject intravenously 25 ml 50 per cent sodium thiosulphate very slowly.

5. If poisoning is due to ingestion, in addition to the above, gastric aspiration and lavage (p. 23) should be given and 300 ml 25 per cent sodium thiosulphate should be left in the stomach.

When severe poisoning has occurred and the amounts of circulating cyanmethaemoglobin and thiocyanate are high, the regimen may need to be repeated using half the original doses of sodium nitrite and sodium thiosulphate.

The patient should be kept resting for at least two days following recovery in order that any anoxic damage, especially to the heart, may be assessed.

Benzene (Benzol)

Benzene is a colourless, volatile liquid with a pleasant smell and is present in many commercial solvents and paint removers. Poisoning usually occurs following inhalation, but may also occur after accidental or intentional ingestion of the liquid.

Clinical Features

Symptoms are mainly related to disturbance of the central nervous system. There is usually initial excitement and restlessness followed by general central nervous depression particularly of the respiratory centre. Death commonly results from respiratory failure, although when the concentration of benzene vapour is high asphyxiation may occur without the other features being apparent.

Treatment

1. In inhalant poisoning, the patient must be removed from exposure to the poison.
2. In ingestant poisoning, gastric aspiration and lavage (p. 23) should be given.
3. Intensive supportive therapy (p. 18) with particular attention to support of respiratory function.

Miscellaneous Organic Solvents

Many readily available commercial substances, such as lacquers, enamels, paint thinners and glues produce vapours of highly volatile organic solvents, which have been used by youngsters to provide 'kicks'[1]. The problem of 'glue sniffing' was first highlighted by Glaser and Massengale in 1962, and, despite efforts by health educators to warn of the dangers of this practice, it remains quite common. Although the toxic features are often relatively mild, deaths have occurred often when a plastic bag is placed over the head to enhance the concentration of the substance inhaled.

Clinical Features

The main effects are on the central nervous system with euphoria and exhilaration but ataxia, slurred speech, drowsiness and coma may result. Habituation and psychological dependence may occur following repeated use.

Treatment

1. Intensive supportive therapy (p. 18) in severe cases.

REFERENCES

Carbon Monoxide
1 Holland, R. A. B. (1965). *J. gen. Physiol.*, **49**, 199.
2 Anderson, R. F., Allensworth, D. C. and De Groot, W. J. (1967). *Ann. intern. Med.*, **67**, 1172.
3 Finck, P. A. (1966). *Milit. Med.*, **131**, 1513.
4 Brucher, J. M. (1967). *Prog. Brain Res.*, **24**, 75.
5 Cosby, R. S. and Bercron, M. (1963). *Amer. J. Cardiol.*, **11**, 93.
6 Long, P. I. (1968). *J. Am. med. Ass.*, **205**, 51.
7 Norman, J. N. and Ledingham, I. McA. (1967). *Prog. Brain Res.*, **24**, 101.

Kerosene and Other Petroleum Distillates
1 Sub-committee on Accidental poisoning. Co-operative kerosene poisoning study. (1962). *Pediatrics*, **29**, 648.
2 Baldachin, B. J. and Melmed, R. N. (1964). *Brit. med. J.*, **2**, 28.

Carbon Tetrachloride
1 Sasame, H. A., Castro, J. A. and Gillette, J. R. (1968). *Biochem. Pharmac.*, **17**, 1759.
2 Rao, K. S. and Recknagel, R. O. (1969). *Expl. molec. Path.*, **10**, 219.

Cyanide
1 Rodkey, F. L. (1967). *Clin. Chem.*, **13**, 2.
2 Schubert, J. and Brill, W. A. (1968). *J. Pharmac. exp. Ther.*, **162**, 352.
3 Williams, R. T. (1959). *Detoxification Mechanisms: The Metabolism and Detoxication of Drugs, Toxic Substances and Other Organic Compounds*, 2nd ed. New York: John Wiley.
4 Lovatt Evans, C. (1964). *Brit. J. Pharmacol.*, **23**, 455.
5 *Brit. med. J.* (1970), **2**, 526.
6 Sheehy, M. and Way, J. L. (1968). *J. Pharmac. exp. Ther.*, **161**, 163.

Miscellaneous Organic Solvents
1 Press, E. and Done, A. K. (1967). *Pediatrics*, **39**, 451.
2 Glaser, H. H. and Massengale, O. N. (1962). *J. Am. med. Ass.*, **181** 300.
3 Leader, *Brit. med. J.* (1971), **2**, 183.

CHAPTER 10

ACUTE POISONING DUE TO COMMON ANALGESICS

Incidence

In adults, acute salicylate poisoning accounts for some 15 per cent of admissions of poisoned patients[1] and in young children, the percentage is even higher. Salicylate, for example, vies with iron preparations as the commonest medicine accidentally taken by infants and toddlers. It is likely to remain a common overdosage as long as aspirin is freely obtainable without prescription. Accidental poisoning may occur in infants and toddlers as a result of injudicious therapy if the dose exceeds 60 mg for each year of age five times per day. Even this dosage schedule should not be continued for more than two days, and adequate fluid intake must be ensured. Poisoning may also arise from the percutaneous absorption of salicylates due to over-enthusiastic use of lotions, ointments and liniments containing salicylic acid. This is the case, especially when extensive areas are being treated and when the skin surface is broken[2].

The mortality in hospital admissions of patients with acute salicylate poisoning is 1-7 per cent[3]. This is, therefore, a dangerous poisoning especially in young children, and in adults serious complications may occur without warning even when patients are carefully monitored[4].

Salicylates

Salicylate poisoning usually arises from an overdose of aspirin itself or some preparation containing it. When compound tablets containing aspirin, phenacetin and codeine are taken in overdose, the most important toxic features are those of salicylism.   The standard aspirin tablet contains 300 mg of acetyl salicylic acid.   Tablets specially prepared to be palatable to children contain smaller amounts, e.g. 230 mg or 100 mg and children often take these in overdose believing them to be sweets.   Methyl salicylate, oil of wintergreen, is very toxic since it is readily absorbed and has a high salicylate content; one teaspoonful is equivalent to 12 standard tablets of aspirin.

Diagnosis and Assessment of Severity

It is a common misconception that patients suffering from acute salicylate poisoning become unconscious.   In adults this is very seldom the case; even drowsiness is unusual and must be regarded as a dangerous sign.   Children react to the effects of salicylate somewhat differently, and drowsiness or even coma is more frequently encountered.

Since the adult patient is likely to be conscious the diagnosis is not difficult.   However, patients frequently exaggerate or understate the number of tablets taken, and although salicylate poisoning is evident, both from the patient's history and the somewhat characteristic clinical findings, a precise assessment of its severity may be difficult to make because the features of salicylism and other symptoms and signs of overdosage may all be present at quite low plasma levels or unimpressive in severe poisoning[5, 6, 7].   This is, therefore, the exceptional occasion when immediate blood analysis is of great value, not only in confirming the diagnosis, but also in assessing the severity of the overdosage.   Quantitative assay can be carried out readily by a doctor in a ward side-room, provided simple equipment is available.   The most simple and satisfactory method is that described on page 14.   A plasma salicylate level of 50 mg/100 ml or more indicates moderate or severe poisoning and intensive forced diuretic therapy must be started.   If however the salicylate has been ingested more than 12 hours previously a considerable quantity of active drug may have been taken up by the tissues and the plasma level may be misleadingly low.   In these circumstances, the determination of arterial blood pH, blood gases and plasma potassium are better indications of the severity of the poisoning.

Clinical Features

The following clinical features of moderate to severe salicylate poisoning will be found in an adult who has ingested about 50 or more standard aspirin tablets, provided, as so often happens, that the patient has not vomited.

Mental alertness and restlessness.

Roaring in the ears, deafness and blurring of vision.

Hyperventilation, the result of a direct stimulating effect on the respiratory centre; both the rate and depth of breathing are increased.

Hyperpyrexia and profuse perspiration.

Epigastric pain and vomiting.

Dehydration due to sweating, vomiting and overbreathing.

Reduced urinary output; the concentrated acid urine contains albumen, and in the initial stages, large numbers of shed renal tubular cells.

The clinical features in children differ somewhat in that they tend to be more sensitive to the toxic effects of salicylate than adults. There is less tendency to mental stimulation and drowsiness commonly occurs.

Laboratory Findings

In all patients there is a mixed acid-base disturbance with respiratory alkalosis and metabolic acidosis. The major complications of this poisoning occur when the acidosis predominates.

ADULTS. In adults, respiratory alkalosis tends to persist for many hours, with a blood pH close to normal despite the increased metabolism and the presence of salicylic acid which might be thought to predispose to acidaemia.

A considerable shift of potassium from extracellular to intracellular space occurs. There is also some increase in the renal excretion of potassium and so hypokalaemia results.

The plasma salicylate level is usually 50 mg/100 ml or more. Hypoprothrombinaemia occurs, but is rarely sufficiently severe to require treatment. Reduction in number and effectiveness of the platelets occurs but seldom results in a bleeding tendency.

CHILDREN. The initial respiratory alkalosis is more quickly followed by the onset of metabolic acidosis, which becomes the main and persistent acid-base abnormality.

Hypokalaemia is less of a problem but hypoglycaemia may be severe.

The plasma salicylate level for moderate poisoning need be no more than 30 mg/100 ml.

Complications

Drowsiness and even unconsciousness may follow sustained acid-base disturbance, especially acidaemia.

Circulatory collapse.

Haemolysis of erythrocytes.

Acute renal failure due to blockage of renal tubules as a result of massive shedding of tubular cells. Permanent renal damage, however, does not seem to follow acute salicylate overdosage.

Pulmonary oedema. Respiratory arrest is a common mode of death.

Treatment

The management of this poisoning is mainly directed towards removal of salicylate from the body[8]. Gastric aspiration and lavage should always be performed irrespective of the time since ingestion (p. 23). Don't procrastinate; it is never too late to aspirate in salicylate!

In mild cases, where there is usually little vomiting, the patients should be simply encouraged to drink freely. In more seriously ill patients (plasma salicylate above 30 mg per 100 ml in children and above 50 mg per 100 ml in adults) positive steps must be taken to increase elimination of the salicylate. Many regimens of treatment have been advocated and include forced water diuresis, forced alkaline diuresis, peritoneal dialysis, haemodialysis or exchange transfusion. Haemodialysis is undoubtedly the most effective method[9], but the necessary facilities are available only in a few centres and even then there is always a significant delay. Although peritoneal dialysis has been used as an alternative, forced diuresis is a simpler and more effective technique. The toxicity of salicylates is due to the amount of free salicylate present and there is general agreement that the urinary excretion of the free form of drug increases in relation to the alkalinity of the urine. Various regimens of treatment to achieve this are available[8, 10, 11], but, with one exception, all may provoke acute changes in acid base and electrolyte balance and require close biochemical monitoring. The most effective method for removing salicylate is forced alkaline diuresis (p. 35), but forced 'cocktail' diuresis (p. 34) has been shown to be almost as effective and causes no biochemical upsets and so laboratory monitoring is unnecessary[8]. This is, therefore, in our view at present the treatment of choice in acute salicylate poisoning. Special equipment is necessary, however, and may not be readily available in general units, in which case forced alkaline diuresis is advised.

Hypertonic solutions and intravenous diuretic drugs have been added to these regimens in an effort to promote a greater flow of urine, but it should be remembered that patients with acute salicylate overdosage may be already severely dehydrated and these preparations are not recommended in this poisoning.

The following protocol is suggested:
1. Heparinized blood should be withdrawn for immediate estimation of the initial plasma salicylate level.
2. Gastric aspiration and lavage should be performed.
3. Forced 'cocktail' diuresis (p. 34) should be started. (See page 33 for contraindications and page 34 for precautions). The plasma salicylate level should be available 15 minutes or so after starting the infusion. If above 50 mg/100 ml the forced diuresis regimen is continued, the aim being

to reduce the serum level to below 35 mg/100 ml when the infusion may be discontinued and the patient encouraged to drink as much as possible. Potassium chloride effervescent may be added to the drinks. If the plasma salicylate level is between 35 and 50 mg/100 ml and features of salicylism are prominent then the forced diuretic regimen should be modified by reducing the infusion rate to 1 litre per hour. The intensive infusion regimen (p. 34) can be safely employed for the following reasons:

Salicylate is frequently the poison of choice with younger persons who can be expected to have healthy kidneys and myocardium.

Severe dehydration is usually present at the outset; indeed no urine may be passed for the first two hours of treatment. Shock is rare in salicylate poisoning.

4. Hypoglycaemia occurs but is corrected in severely ill patients by the dextrose in the diuretic regimen.

5. In severe poisoning over-breathing and profound alkalosis may be so great that physical exhaustion is produced. In these exceptional circumstances curarisation should be considered and breathing maintained by assisted respiration.

6. In very severe poisoning in children, exchange transfusion may be undertaken, provided there is no undue delay in starting this form of treatment.

Bladder catheterisation is very seldom required.

In the potentially lethal situation when the patient has a predominant acidosis, this must be corrected by giving sodium bicarbonate intravenously before giving the full forced diuresis regimen, as these patients are liable to develop acute pulmonary oedema[12].

If forced diuresis cannot be undertaken, peritoneal dialysis (p. 36) or haemodialysis will be effective. It is sometimes said that haemodialysis is mandatory if the salicylate level exceeds 100 mg/100 ml. However, as speed in initiating treatment is so important, it is better to use forced 'cocktail' diuresis in the first place whilst an artificial kidney is being prepared; then if satisfactory diuresis is achieved, the artificial kidney may not be subsequently required.

Forced Alkaline Diuresis in Children

The rate of 'cocktail' infusion in children is 30 ml/kg/hour. Monitoring of serum potassium is important in children. The alkali in the infusion here serves the dual purpose of rendering the urine alkaline and correcting the metabolic acidaemia which is commonly found.

Phenacetin

Numerous proprietary brands of analgesic tablets are mixtures of several drugs and most of them contain aspirin and phenacetin. Toxic effects may result from the misuse of these preparations by lay people treating themselves for minor ailments; self-poisoning episodes also may occur. Acute poisoning is therefore not uncommon and, although the major features of analgesic overdosage are due to the salicylate in the tablets (p. 69) phenacetin toxicity may be a significant factor.

Phenacetin is rapidly absorbed from the alimentary tract and passes quickly from the blood into the tissues. The liver is the main site of metabolism of the drug, and the major metabolite is paracetamol which is excreted in the urine as the glucuronide. A small amount of phenacetin however is converted to paraphenetidin and it is this derivative which is mainly responsible for the methaemoglobinaemia which may be seen in phenacetin overdosage.

As there is a considerable variation in response to phenacetin, and as it is a drug of habituation, assessment of the severity of the poisoning is dependant largely on clinical signs.

Clinical Features

The clinical picture is similar to that which may occur with paracetamol (*vide infra*). For the reasons given above methaemoglobinaemia may also be present.

F

Treatment

The regimen for phenacetin poisoning is similar to that for paracetamol (p. 78).

Paracetamol (Panadol)—Acetaminophen

Because of the substitution of this drug for aspirin in the home medicine cupboard, paracetamol, which is one metabolite of phenacetin, is now becoming a more common cause of overdosage. There is a wide individual variation in tolerance to the drug, but in an adult, serious toxicity usually results from the ingestion of more than 20 tablets each containing 500 mg paracetamol. Liquid preparations for children are also available and contain 120 mg paracetamol in 5 ml. Paracetamol is combined in several tablets with other potent analgesics including propoxyphene, phenylbutazone, aspirin and dihydrocodeine.

Paracetamol is absorbed rapidly from the stomach and upper intestinal tract and is then metabolised quickly in the liver to form glucuronide and sulphate conjugates. Only four per cent is excreted unchanged in the urine[1]. The rate of metabolism is remarkably constant in normal subjects but it has been shown that in patients who develop hepatic damage, which is the most serious and life-threatening toxic effect in this poisoning[2-7], the metabolism is slow[2]. This suggests that the liver damage occurs rapidly after ingestion and that the slow metabolism is a result rather than a cause of the liver damage. The cause of the acute centrilobular necrosis has been shown recently[8-12] to be a highly reactive intermediate metabolite which binds to vital liver cell macromolecules. With therapeutic or small overdosage of paracetamol the amounts of active metabolite formed are rapidly inactivated by conjugation with hepatic glutathione, but toxic doses of paracetamol cause a depletion of this glutathione and if it drops below 30 per cent of normal, hepatic necrosis becomes likely[11]. Administration of glutathione itself is ineffective therapeutically but precursors such as cysteine and cysteamine have been shown to prevent paracetamol-induced hepatic necrosis[11, 12].

Plasma paracetamol levels above 300 μg per ml are very likely to be associated with hepatic damage, which may develop several days after ingestion of the poison. In general, however, the incidence and extent of liver damage cannot readily be related to plasma concentrations of unchanged paracetamol[13]. On the other hand, the plasma paracetamol half-life is very valuable in the early assessment of prognosis. If the plasma paracetamol half-life is greater than four hours, liver damage is likely and if greater than 12 hours, hepatic coma is a real danger[2]. In the assessment of liver function tests and particularly enzyme tests, it is important to take account of additional circumstances such as other existing diseases which might affect liver function and also co-existent poisoning with other drugs. For example, enzyme levels may be elevated in barbiturate coma and yet not indicate significant liver damage and in chronic alcoholics the metabolism of paracetamol may be rapid but the liver may be unduly sensitive to paracetamol toxicity.

Clinical Features

The patient usually is nauseated, pale, sweaty and generally miserable. There may then be some improvement over the next 48 hours prior to the onset of the other features.

HEPATIC DISORDER. An enlarged tender liver, jaundice and other evidence of impaired liver function are not uncommon. Liver damage in this poisoning may be life-threatening and requires careful monitoring.

CARDIOVASCULAR SYSTEM. Hypotension; tachycardia and varied cardiac arrhythmias. Massive overdosage may result in direct toxic damage to the myocardium together with peripheral vasodilatation and severe shock.

CENTRAL NERVOUS SYSTEM. Evidence of cerebral stimulation with excitement may be present. Delirium progressing to central nervous depression and stupor is encountered. The sudden development of coma, either at an early stage or after a period of several days, is usually fatal.

METABOLIC DISORDER. Hypothermia; hyperthermia if the patient develops extensive skin reactions; hypoglycaemia, which may be severe, tends to occur a few days after ingestion. Metabolic acidaemia, which again may be severe.

BLOOD FINDINGS. Acute haemolytic anaemia which, if severe, may result in acute renal failure. Bleeding tendency due to hypoprothrombinaemia and deficiency of other clotting factors.

RESPIRATORY SYSTEM. Dyspnoea; shallow, rapid respiration associated with the acidaemia.

SKIN LESIONS. Erythema and urticaria are quite frequent features, with occasionally mucosal lesions.

Treatment

Various forms of therapy have been advocated for paracetamol overdosage but most have proved ineffective in preventing the hepatic necrosis which is the most serious toxic effect. Antihistamines and corticosteroids, which have been suggested[3], may even increase the toxicity of paracetamol and should not be used[14]. Forced diuresis, charcoal column haemoperfusion and haemodialysis are theoretically effective in removing paracetamol, but in practice the renal excretion of the drug and metabolites is so rapid that these methods of treatment are of very doubtful value for the poisoning *per se*[15, 16, 17]. Ingestion of activated charcoal or cholestyramine[18] is of doubtful value since these substances failed to delay significantly the absorption of paracetamol even when given very quickly after a small dose of the poison[19].

The following regimen is at present the most effective treatment:—

1. Intensive supportive therapy (p. 18).
2. In cases of moderate or severe poisoning in whom the plasma paracetamol half-life is greater than four hours, cysteamine hydrochloride (Sigma, London), 2·0 g intra-

venously over 10 minutes followed by three 400 mg doses in 500 ml of 5 per cent dextrose infused over 4, 8 and 8 hours has been shown to reduce and even prevent liver necrosis[19].

This large dose of cysteamine may cause cutaneous vaso-dilatation, nausea, vomiting and drowsiness which may last 48 hours, but in view of the serious dangers of para-cetamol poisoning, these side-effects are acceptable.

In hepatic failure, where other measures have proved unsatisfactory, exchange blood transfusions and, if facilities are available, pig liver perfusion should be considered.

3. Intravenous infusions of sodium bicarbonate may be necessary to correct the metabolic acidaemia.

4. Intravenous glucose may be required to correct hypo-glycaemia.

5. If haemolysis is severe, corticosteroids and blood trans-fusion may be necessary.

Hypoprothrombinaemia may be corrected by Vitamin K^1 and occasionally other clotting factors may have to be given to correct severe bleeding tendencies.

6. In addition to the usual medical management, haemodialysis may be necessary for acute renal failure.

REFERENCES

Salicylates

1 Sydney Smith, J. and Davison, K. (1971). *Brit. med. J.*, **4**, 412.

2 von Weiss, J. F. and Lever, W. F. (1964). *Arch. Derm.*, **90**, 614.

3 Campbell, H. (1963). In *Salicylates—An International Symposium*, p. 255. London: Churchill.

4 Ghose, R. R. and Joekes, A. M. (1964). *Lancet*, **1**, 1409.

5 Done, A. K. (1965). *J. Am. med. Ass.*, **192**, 770.

6 Brown, S. S., Cameron, J. C. and Matthew, H. (1967). *Brit. med. J.* **1**, 738.

7 Smith, M. J. H. (1966). *The Salicylates*, p. 262. London: Inter-science Publishers.

8 Lawson, A. A. H., Proudfoot, A. T., Brown, S. S., Macdonald, R. H. Fraser, A. G., Cameron, J. C. and Matthew, H. (1969). *Quart. J. med.*, **38**, 31.

9   Maher, J. F. and Schreiner, G. E. (1967). *Trans. Amer. Soc. artificial internal Organs*, **13**, 369.

10   Leader (1969). *Brit. med. J.*, **1**, 3.

11   Leader (1972). *Brit. med. J.*, **1**, 263.

12   Proudfoot, A. T. and Brown, S. S. (1969). *Brit. med. J.*, **2**, 547.

Paracetamol

1   Cummings, A. J., King, M. L. and Martin, B. K. (1967). *Brit. J Pharmac.*, **29**, 150.

2   Prescott, L. F., Wright, N., Roscoe, P. and Brown, S.S. (1971). *Lancet*, **1**, 519.

3   Maclean, D., Peters, T. J., Brown, R. A. G., McCathie, M., Baines, G. F. and Robertson, P. G. C. (1968). *Lancet*, **2**, 849.

4   Pimstone, B. L. and Uys, C. J. (1968). *S. Afr. med. J.*, **42**, 259.

5   Toghill, P. J., Williams, R., Stephens, J. D., and Carroll, J. D. (1969). *Gastroenterology*, **56**, 773.

6   Rose, P. G. (1969). *Brit. med. J.*, **1**, 381.

7   Proudfoot, A. T. and Wright, N. (1970). *Brit. med. J.*, **3**, 557.

8   Mitchell, J. R., Jollow, D. J., Potter, W. Z., Davis, D. C., Gillette, J. R. and Brodie, B. B. (1973). *J. Pharmacol. Exp. Ther.*, **187**, 185.

9.   Jollow, D. J., Mitchell, J. R., Potter, W. Z., Davis, D. C., Gillette, J. R. and Brodie, B. B. (1973). *J. Pharmacol. Exp. Ther.*, **187**, 195.

10   Potter, W. Z., Davis, D. C., Mitchell, J. R., Jollow, D. J., Gillette, J. R. and Brodie, B. B. (1973). *J. Pharmacol. Exp. Ther.*, **187**, 203.

11   Mitchell, J. R., Jollow, D. J., Potter, W. Z., Gillette, J. R. and Brodie, B. B. (1973). *J. Pharmacol. Exp. Ther.*, **187**, 211.

12   Mitchell, J. R., Jollow, D. J., Gillette, J. R. and Brodie, B.B. (1973). *Drug Metabolism and Disposition*, **1**, 418.

13   Brown, S. S., Proudfoot, A. T., Raeburn, J. A., Wright, N. (1970)· *Proc. 7th int. Congr. clin. Chem.* (*Clin. Enzymol. vol.* 2), p. 167. Basle.

14   Nimmo, J., Dixon, M. F. and Prescott, L. F. (1973). *Clin. Toxicol.*, **6**, 75.

15   Nusynowitz, M. L. and Forsham, P. H. (1966). *Amer. J. Med Sci.*, **252**, 429.

16   De Myttenaere, M. H. (1968). In *Proc. 5th Confer. Europ. Dialysis and Transplant Assoc.*, ed. Kerr, D. N. S., Fries D. and Elliot, R. W. p. 320. Amsterdam: Excerpta, Medica.

17   Farid, N. R. Glynn, J. P. and Kerr, D. N. S. (1972). *Lancet*, **2**, 396.

18   Dordoni, B., Willson, R. A., Thompson, R. P. H. and Williams, R. (1973). *Brit. med. J.*, **3**, 86.

19   Prescott, L. F., Newton, R. W., Swainson, C. P., Wright, N., Forrest, A. R. W. and Matthew, H. (1974). *Lancet*, **1**, 588.

CHAPTER 11

ACUTE POISONING WITH ANTIDEPRESSANT DRUGS

Tricyclic Compounds

Acute poisoning with these drugs is common and the incidence is increasing. Inevitably these drugs are prescribed for the very people who are most likely to indulge in self-poisoning or to attempt suicide, and the risk of overdosage is high, especially during the latent period of 14 days or so before many of the tricyclics become effective.

Amitriptyline (Laroxyl, Saroten, Triptafen, Tryptizol), Desipramine (Pertofran), Doxepin (Sinequan), Imipramine (Tofranil), Nortriptyline (Allegron, Aventyl), Protriptyline (Concordin), Trimipramine (Surmontil)

Tricyclic compounds are absorbed rapidly and quickly become firmly protein bound and enter the tissues, so that the blood level is always relatively low. Efficient detoxication occurs in the liver, and very little active drug appears in the urine. Elimination occurs rapidly and 24 hours after ingestion scarcely any of the parent drug remains in the tissues.

Tricyclic antidepressants are toxic in even small amounts but the precise mechanism of action is incompletely known[1]. They act by blockade of acetylcholine-mediated transmitters in the central nervous system and by a powerful anticholinergic effect in the peripheral tissues[2]. The peripheral toxic effects, therefore, resemble those of atropine with resultant tachycardia which, if severe, may cause hypotension. More severe arrhythmias and cardiac conduction defects, which may occur in serious tricyclic overdosage cannot be attributed to the anticholinergic action[3, 4], and these may result from a direct toxic effect on the myocardium or by interference with noradrenaline release from cardiac nerve endings[5].

Clinical Features

Dryness of the mouth.

Dilated pupils.

Atrial and nodal tachycardia and bizarre arrhythmias, e.g. artrio-venticular block, bundle branch block, intraventricular conduction defects and varying ventricular pacemaker.

Depressant effect on the heart with hypotension and ultimate failure or arrest.

Hyper-reflexibility leading to tonic-clonic convulsions, amounting to status epilepticus. Torticollis and ataxia may be pronounced in children.

Hallucinations, usually visual, commonly occur and persist for some days after the other features have disappeared. Pressure of speech is characteristic.

Varying degrees of unconsciousness, but grade IV (p. 18) is rare.

Depression of respiration, which may be severe.

Urinary retention and absent bowel sounds.

These features appear one to two hours after taking the overdose and seldom last for longer than 18-24 hours, but sudden deaths have been reported up to six days after the ingestion of the tricyclic drug and have been presumed to be due to sudden arrhythmias[6, 7, 8]. The cardiac abnormalities are especially prominent and dangerous in children.

Treatment

1. Intensive supportive therapy (p. 18). Gastric aspiration and lavage is of value within 12 hours of ingestion.

   These measures are all that is necessary in the great majority of patients. Even marked sinus tachycardia may be beneficial by virtue of its 'over-drive pacing' effect.

2. Forced diuresis, peritoneal dialysis and haemodialysis are *not* effective in view of the firm tissue binding of these drugs and the very low blood levels.

3. Physostigmine salicylate will abolish the central nervous system effects and will counteract some of the cardiac effects. This anticholinesterase is preferable to neostigmine or prostigmine, which were previously advocated for the treatment of this poisoning, because it readily crosses the blood-brain barrier and is short-acting[9, 10]. Repeat doses may be given, therefore, with greater safety. Physostigmine salicylate (1-3 mg) is given slowly over two minutes by intravenous injection. The effects are usually dramatic with marked improvement in both neurological and cardiac features within 10 minutes, but, if necessary, a second injection may be given after ten minutes. ECG monitoring is desirable. Atrophine sulphate injection should be kept available to counteract any side-effects which may occur from the physostigmine.

4. If the arrhythmia cannot be controlled by physostigmine and is serious, 40 mEq. sodium bicarbonate intravenously may prove effective [11, 12]. The β-adrenergic blocking drug, propranolol, has also been used with success[3, 10]. Digitalis should be avoided as it may increase the heart block and conduction defects[10, 12].

5. Cardiac arrest may occur and require conventional treatment.

6. Hypotension is best treated with plasma expanders. Metaraminol should not be used.

7. If physostigmine fails to control convulsions, diazepam (Valium) 10 mg intravenously is the treatment of choice[10]. If diazepam is ineffective, sodium phenobarbitone 200 mg intramuscularly should be given.

Prognosis

In an adult a dose exceeding 1 g is likely to give rise to serious poisoning. If the patient can be tided over the first 18 hours, and knowing that the drug will largely be metabolised in 24 hours, survival is highly probable. However, sudden death a few days after apparent recovery has been claimed, but the evidence is very slender.

Monoamine Oxidase Inhibitors

This group of drugs is less frequently used in the treatment of depressive illness and so they are an uncommon cause of acute poisoning. The clinical features of acute toxicity are, however, striking, and important precautions must be taken in treatment. The onset of acute toxic effects following over-dosage may be delayed by up to 12 hours. Patients may present with toxic effects due to these drugs either because of acute overdosage *per se*, or because of interactions which may occur when the drugs are given in therapeutic dosage but in association with certain other drugs or with particular items of diet. These effects are dangerous and may even result in death[1].

Cerebral excitation, which may be followed by coma and severe hyperthermia, occurs when monoamine oxidase (MAO) inhibitors are combined with morphine or other opium alkaloids, with anaesthetics and antihistamines, with imipramine and its congeners, anti-parkinsonian drugs, reserpine or methyldopa[2, 3]. The action of guanethidine may be antagonised, whilst with other hypotensive agents, such as pheno-thiazines and thiazide diuretics, the hypotensive effects may be enhanced. The association of monoamine oxidase in-hibitors with sympathomimetic drugs such as amphetamine, ephedrine, noradrenaline and adrenaline evokes adverse reactions whicn include hypertensive crises and in a proportion subarachnoid haemorrhage. There is also a well recognised association of toxicity with eating certain cheeses, especially Cheddar, Camembert and Stilton; broad beans and Marmite have also been incriminated as precipitating factors. This is particularly the case in patients treated with tranylcypro-mine[4, 5]. The substance in the cheeses which has been im-plicated as the provocative factor is tyramine[6]. Monoamine oxidase inhibitors also appear to prolong and potentiate the actions of anaesthetics, opiates, barbiturates, alcohol and insulin. All these possibilities result in severe upset to the patient and although there may have been no actual over-dosage of any one substance they may truly be regarded as acute poisonings.

Monoamine oxidase inhibitors are both readily absorbed from the gastrointestinal tract and rapidly excreted as the acid metabolite but their effects are prolonged due to irreversible inhibition of the enzyme. Enzyme function takes weeks to return to normal. Hydrazine MAO inhibitors must first undergo cleavage before the drug becomes active. Non-hydrazine MAO inhibitors can combine directly with the enzyme.

Clinical Features

DRUG AND FOOD INTERACTION

Headache.

Fever.

Hypertensive crisis with possible intracranial haemorrhage, or hypotension.

Cerebral excitation and convulsions.

Loss of consciousness.

Cardiac arrhythmias.

ACUTE OVERDOSAGE OF MONOAMINE OXIDASE INHIBITORS

Agitation.

Hallucinations.

Tachycardia.

Hyper-reflexia.

Sweating.

Hyperthermia or hypothermia.

Convulsions.

Hypotension or hypertension.

Urinary retention.

Spasticity.

Treatment

The basic principles of intensive supportive therapy (p. 18) should be followed but there are a number of very important precautions which *must* be observed.

1. Metaraminol (Aramine) and other sympathomimetic agents must *not* be given in the treatment of hypotension. Intra-

venous infusion of plasma expanders should be used. Severe shock should be treated by hydrocortisone (100 mg intravenously) every six hours.

2. Chloropromazine is the drug of choice to combat cerebral excitement but if convulsions occur then sodium pheno-barbitone 300 mg intramuscularly should be given.

3. Hypertensive crises should be treated by using a short-acting hypotensive agent such as pentolinium (0·25 mg intramuscularly) or phentolamine 5 mg intravenously followed by phenoxybenzamine 100 mg in 200 ml 5 per cent dextrose intravenously over 90 minutes.

4. Hyperthermia may be corrected by cooling with a damp sheet and a fan, but if severe, chlorpromazine 100 mg intramuscularly is highly effective.

5. Forced diuresis and peritoneal dialysis are probably ineffective but haemodialysis is of value in very severely poisoned patients.

Lithium

Lithium carbonate (Camcolit, Priadel) is now being used with increasing frequency in the treatment of manic depression, hence overdosage is likely[1, 2].

Lithium is a monovalent cation and belongs to the group of alkali metals together with sodium and potassium. It is readily absorbed from the gut and is not bound to plasma proteins. It passes readily from the blood into the tissues and rapidly equilibrates, but there may be considerable accumulation in liver, muscle, brain and kidney. It is not metabolised and excretion is mainly through the kidney in competition with sodium ions. The therapeutic index is low. Features of toxicity are particularly liable to occur in patients who are being treated with lithium and who are then given a regimen liable to promote salt depletion such as dietary salt restriction and diuretics[3]. Also during pregnancy the renal clearance of lithium increases markedly and the plasma levels of the drug may fall, but after delivery the reverse happens rapidly and the blood levels may reach toxic levels even without any change in the dosage given[4].

Clinical Features

Severe thirst, polyuria, vomiting and diarrhoea.
Drowsiness leading to impaired consciousness.
Tremor, hypertonicity and convulsions.
Blood level above 1·5 mEq/litre indicates toxicity although the therapeutic range is 0·7-1·3 mEq/litre[2, 5].

Treatment

1. Intensive supportive therapy (p. 18).
2. Forced alkaline diuresis (p. 35), but in view of associated changes in sodium and potassium balance with this poisoning close monitoring of plasma electrolytes is mandatory.
3. If hypertonicity occurs convulsions are to be anticipated and phenobarbitone 300 mg should be given intramuscularly. Pentothal may be required to control established convulsions.
4. Peritoneal and haemodialysis (p. 36) are likely to be effective, but may require to be repeated owing to lithium being withdrawn from tissue accumulation. In our experience, however, supported by laboratory data, forced diuresis is as effective as peritoneal or haemodialysis.

REFERENCES

Tricyclic Compounds

1 Servis, T. L., Ott, J. E., Teitelbaum, D. T. and Libscomb, W. (1971). *Clin. Toxicol.*, 4(3), 451.
2 Jarvick, M. E. (1970). In *The Pharmacological Basis of Therapeutics*, ed. Goodman, L. S. and Gilman, A., 4th ed., p. 186. New York: Collier.
3 Barnes, R. J., Kong, S. M. and Wu, R. W. Y. (1968). *Brit. med. J.*, 3, 222.
4 Freeman, J. W., Mundy, G. R., Beattie, R. R. and Ryan, C. (1969). *Brit. med. J.*, 2, 610.
5 Sigg, E. B., Osborne, M. and Korol, B. (1963). *J. Pharmacol. Expl. Therap.*, 141, 237.

6 Steel, C. M., O'Duffy, J. and Brown, S. S. (1967). *Brit. med. J.*, **3**, 663.

7 Master, A. B. (1967). *Brit. med. J.*, **3**, 886.

8 Brackenridge, R. G., Peters, T. J. and Watson, J. M. (1968). *Scot. med. J.*, **13**, 208.

9 Duvoisin, R. C. and Katz, R. (1968). *J. Am. med. Ass.*, **206**, 1963.

10 Hall, R. (1970). *National Clearinghouse for Poison Control Centres Bulletin* (May-June).

11 Frejaville, J. P., Nicaise, A. M., Christoforov, B., Staer, J. D., Pébay-Peyroula, F. and Gaultier, M. (1966). *Bull. Soc. Med. Hop. Paris*, **117**, 1151.

12 Prudhommeaux, J. L., Lechat, P. and Auclair, M. C. (1968). *Therapie*, **23** 675.

Monoamine Oxidase Inhibitors

1 Jarvik, M. E. (1967). In *The Pharmacological Basis of Therapeutics*, ed. Goodman, L.S. and Gilman, A., 3rd ed., p. 191. New York: Collier.

2 Crisp, A. H., Hays, P. and Carter, A. (1961). *Lancet*, **1**, 17.

3 Moser, M., Brodoff, B., Bakan, H. and Miller, A. (1961). *J. Am. med. Ass.*, **176**, 276.

4 Davies, E. B. (1963). *Lancet*, **2**, 691.

5 Kraines, S. H. (1964). *J. Am. med. Ass.*, **188**, 612.

6 Asatoor, A. M., Levi, A. J. and Milne, M. D. (1963). *Lancet*, **2**, 733.

Lithium

1 Schou, M. and Baastrup, P. C. (1967). *J. Am. med. Ass.*, **201**, 696.

2 Saran, B. M. and Gaind, R. (1973). *Clin. Toxicol.*, **6** (2), 257.

3 Schou, M., Amdisen, A. and Steenstrup, O. R. (1973). *Brit. med. J.*, **2**, 137.

4 Weinstein, M. R. and Goldfield, M. D. (1970). *J. Am. med. Ass.*, **214**, 1325.

5 Schou, M., Amdisen, A. and Baastrup, P. C. (1971). *Brit. J. Hospital Med.*, **6**, 53.

CHAPTER 12

ACUTE POISONING WITH TRANQUILLISER DRUGS

The term 'tranquilliser' was originally applied to drugs with the ability to sedate without causing hypnosis or anaesthesia. With the introduction of new preparations and with increased clinical experience of these drugs, this concept must be broadened to include antipsychotic action and effects on behaviour disturbance. A number of other terms, such as 'antiphobic', 'psycholeptic' and 'psychotropic' have been coined to describe the complex actions of this group of drugs. It can still be claimed, however, that 'tranquilliser' is the most generally accepted description.

The group now includes many preparations, with widely differing pharmacological actions. They are prescribed very frequently and, in some quarters, with gay abandon. For this reason, and also as these drugs are intended for people already with psychological abnormality, it is not surprising that there is a high incidence of acute overdosage.

The Phenothiazines

The most effective tranquillisers are in this group, and they tend to be the drugs most frequently prescribed in the treatment of psychoses.

The phenothiazines are well absorbed from the gastro-intestinal tract and from parenteral sites. About 70 per cent of an administered dose is rapidly taken up by the liver and there is a very active enterohepatic circulation. The biological half-life of the phenothiazines is very long, and various metabolites or even free drug may be detected in the urine 6 to 12 months after treatment is stopped. Approximately half of the metabolites of the phenothiazines are found in the urine and the remainder in the faeces. Even in severe overdosage the blood levels of these drugs are very low and are measured in micrograms per 100 ml.

Clinical Features

These have been reviewed in detail by McKown and his colleagues[1].

Tolerance usually develops on prolonged therapy with these drugs. This possibility must therefore be considered in the assessment of the poisoned patient.

CENTRAL NERVOUS SYSTEM. Loss of consciousness.

Parkinsonism[2, 3], with muscle rigidity, tremor and increased limb reflexes.

Dyskinesia, including torticollis, facial grimacing, abnormal eye movements and possibly oculogyric crisis.

Akathisia, with marked restlessness. In severe poisoning convulsions may occur. These extrapyramidal effects are particularly marked in young children and may last for a prolonged time[3].

CARDIOVASCULAR SYSTEM. *Hypotension*, which may be severe, and is due to both direct and indirect effects of the drug, viz.:

(a) Direct depressant effect on the myocardium.

(b) Direct vasodilating effect on the peripheral circulation.

(c) Inhibition of centrally mediated pressor reflexes.

(d) Peripheral and ganglionic adrenergic blockade.

Tachycardia which results from the lowered peripheral resistance, leading to hypotension.

Arrhythmias[4]. Various arrhythmias may develop with a tendency to be resistant to the usual methods of treatment. Cardiac arrest is uncommon but may occur. ECG changes: prolongation of the Q-T interval and blunting of the T waves are common.

RESPIRATORY SYSTEM. Except in the most severe overdosage respiratory depression is uncommon.

METABOLIC DISORDERS. Effects on temperature. Hypothermia is most common and may be severe, but on occasions, the patient may be slightly hyperthermic.

Toxicological Diagnosis

As the blood levels in this poisoning are very low analysis of the urine is more likely to be of diagnostic value than that of the blood (p. 14).

Treatment

1. Intensive supportive therapy should form the basis of treatment of acute overdosage with the phenothiazines (p. 18).
2. Methods of treatment designed to increase removal of these drugs, such as haemodialysis are ineffective.
3. Dyskinesia should be treated by repeated injections of benztropine mesylate (Cogentin) 2 mg intravenously.
4. Convulsions are best controlled by diazepam (Valium) 10 mg intravenously supplemented by sodium phenobarbitone 200 mg intramuscularly.
5. As phenothiazines are adrenergic blocking agents, they provide some protection against the deleterious effects of circulatory shock. In particular, in addition to having a direct diuretic action there is evidence that they prevent the fall of renal blood flow even when the systemic blood pressure is low. For these reasons strenuous efforts need not be made to elevate the blood pressure provided the patient is producing urine.
6. Attempts should be made to treat cardiac arrhythmias with the appropriate drug such as lignocaine, digoxin, procainamide and propranolol. If there is accompanying severe hypotension, this should be corrected, if possible with plasma expanders, as this makes the arrhythmias more easily corrected.

Rauwolfia Alkaloids

Reserpine and the rauwolfia alkaloids are used primarily as hypotensive agents, but have certain properties in common

G

with the phenothiazines. They are occasionally used in the treatment of psychoses when response to phenothiazines has been inadequate. Even in small doses, the rauwolfia alkaloids are notorious for causing acute depression, which may precipitate suicidal tendencies, but overdosage with these preparations is uncommon.

Rauwolfia alkaloids are absorbed readily from the gastrointestinal tract and from parenteral sites, and are probably rapidly taken up by depot fat. These drugs deplete stores of catecholamines and 5-hydroxytryptamine in many tissues including brain, heart, blood vessels and the adrenal medulla. The consequent clinical effects tend to be rather slow in onset, but may persist for some days after urinary excretion of the drug and its various metabolites has ceased.

Clinical Features

GENERAL. Flushed skin; dry mouth; nasal congestion.

CENTRAL NERVOUS SYSTEM. Loss of consciousness; parkinsonism; chorea and cerebellar disorder may occur.

CARDIOVASCULAR SYSTEM. Hypotension which may persist for some days following acute overdosage. Bradycardia; arrhythmias—usually ectopic beats; acute congestive failure especially in patients with previous myocardial or renal disease, as the result of acute sodium and water retention.

ALIMENTARY SYSTEM. Abdominal cramps and diarrhoea.

RESPIRATORY SYSTEM. Respiratory depression may be severe and is the usual mode of death in this poisoning.

Treatment

The general principles of treatment described for the phenothiazines are applicable to acute overdosage of rauwolfia alkaloids. Diuretics however should be used in preference to digoxin if congestive cardiac failure occurs, as digoxin would intensify the bradycardia and make arrhythmias more frequent. Severe hypotension is here more likely to result in renal damage than in the acute poisoning with phenothiazines and so requires treatment with metaraminol and, if necessary, plasma expanders (p. 21).

Benzodiazepins

CHLORDIAZEPOXIDE (LIBRIUM), DIAZEPAM (VALIUM), NITRA-ZEPAM (MOGADON). These compounds are in frequent use as mild tranquillisers and night sedatives. They are also commonly prescribed with antidepressant drugs for the management of certain depressive illnesses, and so are often available to a group of the population who are prone to take an overdosage of drugs. Acute overdosage is therefore common and in some centres drugs in this group are the commonest ingested, replacing the barbiturates. Fortunately the effects are surprisingly mild[1, 2].

Absorption of benzodiazepins from the gastrointestinal tract tends to be rather slow; several hours elapse before peak blood levels are reached after oral administration. Plasma levels then fall slowly and the excretion of the drug in the urine may continue for several days. Less than 5 per cent of the ingested dose is recovered in the urine as unaltered drug.

Clinical Features

The effects are surprisingly mild and there is no authenticated death from these drugs[3, 4]. As many as 100 tablets of nitraze-pam may be taken with remarkably little effect.

CENTRAL NERVOUS SYSTEM. Drowsiness with possible coma in very rare instances. Dizziness, ataxia and slurred speech.

CARDIOVASCULAR SYSTEM. Rarely, mild hypotension.

RESPIRATORY SYSTEM. Respiratory depression occurs infrequently and is not severe.

Treatment

1. Intensive supportive therapy (p. 18) is all that will be required.

2. Forced diuresis, peritoneal dialysis and haemodialysis are *not* effective and in any event would never be indicated as the patient is never more than drowsy.

Carbamates

The carbamate group of compounds include (meprobamate (Equanil, Mepavlon, Miltown), ethinamate (Valmid, Valmidate) and methylpentynol carbamate (Oblivon-C).

MEPROBAMATE

On account of being widely prescribed for agitated, anxious or distressed patients, meprobamate is occasionally taken in overdosage in Britain, but, more commonly in the United States. Surprisingly there is little reliable information either as to what constitutes a dangerous amount taken or as to the blood levels associated with features of overdosage, or the efficacy of various forms of treatment. This information may be lacking because severe poisoning or a fatal outcome is seldom seen[1, 2].

Meprobamate is quickly absorbed and fairly rapidly metabolised—much more so than barbiturates or glutethimide. Even after a large overdosage, most of the drug will be excreted or inactivated within 24 hours.

Deep coma is to be anticipated if the plasma level is over 10 mg/100 ml. Levels of 20 mg/100 ml have been encountered in patients habituated to the drug. Consciousness may be retained with a plasma level of up to 5 mg/100 ml.

Clinical Features

CENTRAL NERVOUS SYSTEM. Varying degree of unconsciousness. Muscle weakness and inco-ordination. Nystagmus.

RESPIRATORY SYSTEM. Respiratory depression.

CARDIOVASCULAR SYSTEM. Hypotension. Petechial haemorrhages due to capillary toxic damage.

METABOLIC DISORDERS. Hypothermia.

LABORATORY FINDINGS. A plasma level greater than 5 mg per 100 ml indicates overdosage.

Drug dependence may be present if the patient has been treated for some time with large doses of meprobamate. Withdrawal features may therefore be seen, such as convulsions.

Treatment

1. Intensive supportive therapy (p. 18) is usually all that is required[1].
2. Forced osmotic diuresis in severely poisoned patients (p. 35). The severity of the poisoning is judged on the clinical state of the patient and in severe cases the plasma level of meprobamate is usually about 20 mg per 100 ml. When forced diuresis is contraindicated on clinical grounds (p. 33) haemodialysis should be used[1].
3. Peritoneal dialysis is *not* effective.

Prognosis

The metabolism of meprobamate is so rapid that within 24 hours even a very severely poisoned patient will regain consciousness with intensive supportive therapy only. Methods to hasten the removal of the drug are therefore very seldom required and should be reserved for poisoned patients who do not respond rapidly to intensive supportive therapy.

ETHINAMATE

The effects of overdosage with ethinamate are similar to those caused by methylpentynol carbamate and the treatment is the same.

METHYLPENTYNOL CARBAMATE

Acute poisoning with this drug is uncommon. The toxic effects and treatment are referred to on page 102.

REFERENCES

Phenothiazines

1 McKown, C. H., Verhulst, H. L. and Crotty, J. J. (1965). *J. Am. med. Assoc.*, **185**, 425.

2 Angle, C. R., McIntire, M. S. and Zettermann, R. (1968) *Clin. Toxicol.*, **1**, 16.

3 Angle, C. R. and McIntire, M. S. (1968). *J. Pediatrics*, **73**, 124.

4 Giles, T. D. and Modlin, R. K. (1968). *J. Am. med. Assoc.*, **205**, 108.

Benzodiazepins

1 Matthew, H., Proudfoot, A. T., Aitken, R. C. B., Raeburn, J. A. and Wright, N. (1969). *Brit. med. J.*, **3**, 23.

2 Barraclough, B. M. (1974). *Lancet*, **1**, 57.

3 Matthew, H. (1974). *Lancet*, **1**, 224.

4 Lader, M. H. (1973). *Brit. J. Hospital Med.*, **1**, 79.

Meprobamate

1 Maddock, R. K. and Bloomer, H. A. (1967). *J. Am. med. Ass.*, **201**, 999.

2 Lader, M. H. (1973). *Brit. J. Hospital Med.*, **1**, 79.

CHAPTER 13

NON-BARBITURATE HYPNOTICS

There is constant endeavour to produce new hypnotic preparations as satisfactory alternatives to the barbiturates. Non barbiturate hypnotics are frequently presented to the medical profession as safe and non-habit forming, but from the very nature of their action it is unlikely that hypnotic drugs can ever be completely safe or relied upon not to induce dependence. An exception to this (p. 93) is nitrazepam (Mogadon).

Glutethimide (Doriden)

In Britain this drug is less commonly taken in overdosage than in America. Certain clinical features of the poisoning and aspects of its treatment warrant description.

Glutethimide is poorly soluble in water but much more so in alcohol. The ingestion of alcohol along with the tablets, therefore, greatly facilitates absorption from the stomach. Being readily soluble also in fat, it is rapidly stored in tissues, and then only slowly released into the bloodstream. It is metabolised in the liver and it has recently been shown by Fischer[1] that a hydroxy metabolite rises to high levels in the plasma as the plasma glutethimide levels are declining. This metabolite was shown to be at least as toxic to mice as the parent drug. This probably explains why plasma levels of glutethimide do not correlate with the clinical course. Fluctuation of the level of unconsciousness so often seen in glutethimide poisoning could also be explained on the basis of the production of a toxic metabolite.

Clinical Features

The general features of overdosage are similar to those of

barbiturate poisoning (p. 51) but certain differences require emphasis:

CENTRAL NERVOUS SYSTEM. The depth of coma may vary considerably, being interspersed with periods of partial arousal. This fluctuation occurs in overdosage with several hypnotic drugs, but is most marked in glutethimide poisoning. The exact cause is uncertain but factors to be considered include the production of a toxic metabolite, the erratic absorption from the intestine as shock improves, the release from tissue stores and the significant anticholinergic action of the drug.

Episodes of sudden apnoea may occur, which are probably due to acute raised intracranial pressure as papilloedema is often present at the time[2].

The pupils tend to be dilated and unresponsive to light.

CARDIOVASCULAR SYSTEM. Hypotension may be severe and disproportionate to the degree of unconsciousness. Myocardial damage due to a direct toxic effect of the drug may also occur.

LABORATORY FINDING;. A plasma level of 3 mg per 100 ml or more is associated with severe poisoning unless the patient is tolerant to the drug.

Severe and persistent acidosis may occur.

Treatment

1. Intensive supportive therapy as detailed (p. 18). When gastric aspiration and lavage is undertaken the lavage fluid should consist of a mixture of equal quantities of castor oil and water shaken together; 50 ml of castor oil should be left in the stomach on completion of lavage.

2. Acidosis should be corrected and special attention given to the possibility of its recurrence.

3. Sudden episodes of apnoea can be prevented (or if present treated) by giving 500 ml 20 per cent mannitol intravenously over 20 minutes followed by 500 ml 5 per cent dextrose over the next four hours. This should be given where there is any suspicion of acute raised intracranial pressure.

4. Although commonly advocated for the treatment of this poisoning, haemodialysis is relatively ineffective even in serious overdoses, as the recovery of active drug will not exceed more than one or two tablets[3]. There is evidence, however, that the addition of soya bean oil to the dialysing fluid will augment the amount of drug recovered but even then the amount of drug recovered is probably not significant. It is important that the dialysis should be continued for at least two hours after the patient regains consciousness, otherwise there may be a relapse into deep coma on the subsequent release of drug from depot fat.
5. Forced diuresis and peritoneal dialysis are *not* effective[4].
6. Analeptic drugs, such as bemegride (Megimide) are of *no* value. It should be remembered that their presence may interfere with the identification and assay of glutethimide in blood.
7. Withdrawal features resembling delirium tremens are uncommon.

Prognosis

The mortality rate from glutethimide poisoning has been reported to be as high as 70 per cent after the ingestion of 12 g glutethimide. In other series, it has been about 20 per cent, but we agree with Chazan and Garella[5] and Wright and Roscoe[4] that the mortality should not be greater than 2 per cent using conservative treatment alone.

Methaqualone

This quinazolone compound has been extensively used on the European continent for a number of years. The most popular brand preparation in the United States is Quaalude, but in Britain the largest manufacturers have recently withdrawn their preparation. It is, however, still available compounded with diphenhydramine as Mandrax. A survey in Edinburgh in 1970 showed that 10 per cent of all acute ingestant poisonings were due to overdosage with Mandrax. This figure has now been halved. Addiction and misuse are common[1]. The antihistamine component does not appear to contribute significantly to its toxicity.

Methaqualone is readily absorbed after oral administration, and the hypnotic effect is manifest within 30 minutes. Only 2 per cent unchanged drug is excreted in the urine.

The metabolic, kinetic, pharmacological and clinical features have been extensively reviewed by Brown and Goenechea[2].

Clinical Features

CENTRAL NERVOUS SYSTEM. Depression of consciousness which may be severe. Hypertonia with increased limb reflexes and myoclonia. Extensor plantar responses and papilloedema may be found and convulsions may occur.

CARDIOVASCULAR SYSTEM. Tachycardia is common. In severe cases acute myocardial damage may result even in patients without previously known coronary vascular disease.

RESPIRATORY SYSTEM. There is a danger of acute pulmonary oedema but severe respiratory depression is rare.

BLOOD FINDINGS. Bleeding tendencies may be apparent. Clotting factor deficiencies are sometimes found but the significance of this in relation to the haemorrhagic tendency noted is obscure.

LABORATORY FINDINGS. Potentially dangerous intoxication is indicated by blood levels of methaqualone greater than 3 mg per cent in patients who do not have tolerance to the drug. This develops with prolonged therapy.

The pyramidal signs described are striking and offer a useful indication of this particular type of overdosage. Such signs do occur in other poisonings for example, by tricyclic compounds, but methaqualone intoxication should always be suspected when these features are present[3].

Treatment

1. Intensive supportive therapy (p. 18) has proved satisfactory for this type of poisoning.

2. Forced diuresis is not effective as only 2 per cent of active drug is excreted in the urine and should *not* be used because of the tendency to pulmonary oedema and possible myocardial damage. Even haemodialysis is ineffective unless in gravely ill patients in whom the blood level of methaqualone is greater than 10 mg per 100 ml[4].

Chloral and its Congeners

A number of very effective drugs owe their central depressant actions to the fact that they give rise in the body to the active compound trichlorethanol. In addition, to chloral itself, the most commonly prescribed preparations of this type are dichloralphenazone (Welldorm) and triclofos (Tricloryl).

Acute poisoning with these preparations may occur by simple overdosage, but sometimes chloral is mixed with alcohol to provide the well-known 'knock-out drops', popularly known as 'Mickey Finn'. This may be administered with criminal intent.

Chloral and its congeners are readily absorbed from the gastrointestinal tract, and become widely distributed throughout the body. The active principle, trichlorethanol, is formed by reductive processes; detoxication occurs both by conjugation, to give the glucuronide, and by oxidation to trichloracetic acid. The metabolites, with trichlorethanol itself, are excreted in the urine in variable amounts during a period of one to two days after a single dose.

Clinical Features

As chloral evokes a considerable variation in response from one patient to another estimated potentially fatal doses are misleading.

Acute overdosage of chloral hydrate in general resembles acute barbiturate poisoning but, in addition, the patient may complain of a retrosternal 'burning' sensation; gastric irritation may cause vomiting. On occasions, jaundice may develop after the initial effects of the overdosage have resolved. Albuminuria may also be found as a result of renal damage.

Treatment

Basic symptomatic treatment as described under Intensive Supportive Therapy (p. 18), is almost always entirely adequate. In very severe poisoning, forced diuresis (p. 33) or dialysis (p. 36) may be considered.

Tertiary Alcohols

Acetylenic tertiary alcohols are quite potent central nervous depressants. Two in particular are commonly prescribed, i.e. methylpentynol (Oblivon) and ethchlorvynol (Arvynol).

METHYLPENTYNOL

This is a mild soporific which is readily absorbed following oral administration. It is an uncommon cause of acute poisoning, but in high therapeutic doses, a cumulative effect may develop over a few days.

Clinical Features

The signs and symptoms of this poisoning resemble inebriation with alcohol. The patient may be either very tearful or else highly elated. Conjunctival injection, nystagmus and double vision are all common. Drowsiness, mental confusion and ataxia occur.

Treatment

Supportive measures are all that are required.

ETHCHLORVYNOL (PLACIDYL, ARVYNOL)

This preparation is also readily absorbed from the gastro-intestinal tract. A peak blood level is reached about one and a half hours after ingestion of a therapeutic dose, but none can be detected after three hours. Its effects are potentiated if taken in association with alcohol, and loss of consciousness may then persist for many days. Habituation and tolerance occur in patients on continuing therapy, and withdrawal symptoms may occur if the drug is stopped.

Clinical Features

A helpful diagnostic sign is the characteristic pungent aromatic odour of the breath and of material removed by gastric lavage. The clinical features resemble those of other hypnotic drugs but are often severe and prolonged. Deep coma with sometimes fluctuation in level, severe respiratory depression, bradycardia with hypotension and hypothermia are typical of this poisoning. Respiratory infection seems to be commoner than can be explained by the duration of coma and may be due to a direct toxic effect on the lungs.

Treatment

Intensive supportive therapy with particular attention to respiration (p. 18) is usually all that is required. Confusion has arisen regarding the efficacy of forced diuresis in this poisoning. Certain analytical methods commonly used measure inactive metabolites as well as the parent drug, resulting in a falsely high estimate of the amount of drug recovered. Gibson and Wright[2] have shown conclusively that haemodialysis is effective in removing worthwhile amounts of active drug in severely poisoned patients; the amount recovered by forced diuresis is negligible.

NITRAZEPAM (MOGADON)

This is a commonly prescribed hypnotic but as it belongs to the benzodiazepin group of drugs the features of poisoning due to this compound are described on page 93.

REFERENCES

Glutethimide
1 Personal communication (1974).
2 Linton, A. L. (1966). *Scot. med. J.*, **11,** 295.

3 Chazan, J. A. and Cohen, J. J. (1969). *J. Am. med. Ass.*, **208** (5), 837.
4 Wright, N. and Roscoe, P. (1970). *J. Am. med. Ass.*, **214** (9), 1702.
5 Chazan, J. A. and Garella, S. (1971). *Arch. intern. med.*, **128**, 215.

Methaqualone
1 Forrest, J. A. H. and Tarala, R. A. (1973). *Brit. med. J.*, **4**, 136.
2 Brown, S. S. and Goenechea, S. (1973). *Clin. Pharmacol. and Therap.*, **14** (3), 314.
3 Matthew, H., Proudfoot, A. T., Brown, S. S. and Smith, A. C. A. (1968). *Brit. med. J.*, **2**, 101.
4 Proudfoot, A. T., Noble, J., Nimmo J., Brown, S. S. and Cameron, J. C. (1968). *Scot. med. J.*, **13**, 232.

Ethchlorvynol
1 Teehan, B. P., Maher, J. F., Carey, J. H., Flynn, P. D., Schreiner, G. E. (1970). *Ann. intern. med.*, **72**, 875.
2 Gibson, P. F. and Wright, N. (1972). *J. Pharmac. Science*, **61** (2), 169.

CHAPTER 14

NON-BARBITURATE ANTICONVULSANTS

Epileptics are frequently psychologically disturbed and are therefore more prone than members of the general population to self-poisoning and even, on occasions, to true attempted suicide. For this reason acute overdosage of the non-barbiturate anticonvulsants is common.

Hydantoin Compounds

PHENYTOIN (EPANUTIN)

This is commonly prescribed for the treatment of grand mal epilepsy. There is good absorption following oral administration, but the onset of action is rather slow and its duration may be quite prolonged, compared with the barbiturates. The liver is the main site of detoxication and several metabolites are excreted in the urine[1].

Clinical Features

CENTRAL NERVOUS SYSTEM. Stimulation and possibly euphoria; vertigo; headache; tremor; loss of consciousness; cerebellar ataxia and nystagmus, which may last for several days[2].

GASTROINTESTINAL SYSTEM. Nausea and vomiting. Haematemesis occasionally occurs and may be severe.

RESPIRATORY SYSTEM. Depression of respiration may occur.

The features are usually relatively mild and death rarely results.

Treatment

Intensive supportive therapy (p. 18).

METHOIN (MESONTOIN)

This drug is of similar constitution to phenytoin, but is a more potent substance. Severe toxic effects, such as marked loss of consciousness may result from even a small overdosage of this drug.

PRIMIDONE (MYSOLINE)

This compound is a congener of phenobarbitone and like it, is a commonly prescribed oral anticonvulsant preparation. It is metabolised by oxidative processes, mainly in the liver, which result, in part, in its conversion to phenobarbitone itself. Up to 50 per cent of an ingested dose of primidone may be metabolised to phenobarbitone in this way. Many of its therapeutic and indeed toxic effects probably result from the phenobarbitone formed.

Clinical Features

These are similar to the effects of overdosage with hydantoin drugs (*vide supra*), although loss of consciousness tends to be more marked and to occur at an earlier stage. After recovery from the immediate toxic effects of the drug, the patient may continue to be ataxic and to complain of tremor for some days.

Treatment

1. Intensive supportive therapy (p. 18) is almost always sufficient.
2. In very severe poisoning forced alkaline osmotic diuresis (p. 35) or one of the methods of dialysis (p. 36) should be considered.

Paraldehyde

Paraldehyde is used as a hypnotic and anticonvulsant. It is, on the whole, a very safe drug, but acute poisoning occasionally occurs. If exposed to light or air it decomposes in part to acetaldehyde and other products, and a number of instances of acute poisoning have occurred following the use of samples which have deteriorated in this way.

Paraldehyde is well absorbed from the gastrointestinal tract but as it is very irritant and has an unpleasant taste, the usual route of administration is intramuscular injection. A significant proportion of the drug is excreted through the lungs and this imparts a characteristic smell to the exhaled breath which simplifies diagnosis.

Clinical Features[4]

RESPIRATORY SYSTEM. Rapid, laboured breathing, due to two factors: (a) damage to the lungs by paraldehyde and its metabolic products, and (b) acidosis[5].

After intravenous injection, pulmonary haemorrhage and oedema may occur.

GASTROINTESTINAL SYSTEM. Bleeding from the stomach, nausea and vomiting may be apparent following ingestion.

HEPATIC DISORDER. Acute toxic hepatitis sometimes results.

RENAL DISORDERS. Albuminuria, oliguria and uraemia all may occur.

Treatment

Intensive supportive therapy (p. 18). If hepatic or renal damage is present hydrocortisone (100 mg) intravenously at six-hourly intervals may be of benefit.

Sulthiame (Ospolot)

This drug, used in the treatment of temporal lobe and Jacksonian epilepsy, is a sulphonamide congener with weak carbonic anhydrase activity. Over 80 per cent of the active drug is excreted in the urine.

The effects of even massive overdosage are likely to be short lived with the exception of renal damage, which may result from heavy crystalluria due to excreted drug if the urine is acid[6]. The other clinical features include hyperventilation with consequent acid-base upset, clouding of consciousness with marked unawareness of surroundings, brisk limb reflexes with extensor plantar responses. Catatonia may be evident[7].

Treatment

Intensive supportive therapy (p. 18) is likely to suffice in the majority of patients, the only special feature being the necessity to keep the urine alkaline. In severe poisoning, forced alkaline diuresis (p. 35) will procure rapid excretion of the drug.

DIAZEPAM (VALIUM)

This benzodiazepin drug is commonly used as an anticonvulsant. The features of overdosage are described on p. 93.

REFERENCES

1 Toman, J. E. P. (1970). Drugs effective in convulsive disorders. In *The Pharmacological Basis of Therapeutics*, ed. Goodman, L. S. and Gilman, A, p. 210. New York: Collier.

2 Patel, H. and Crichton, J. U. (1968). *J. Pediat.*, **73**, 676.

3 Lennox, W. G. and Lennox, M. A. (1960). *Epilepsy and Related Disorders*. Boston: Little, Brown & Co.

4 Sharpless, S. K. (1970). Hypnotics and sedatives. In *The Pharmacological Basis of Therapeutics*, ed. Goodman, L. S. and Gilman, A., p. 127. New York: Collier.

5 Beier, L. S., Pitts, W. H. and Gonick, H. C. (1963). *Ann. intern. med.*, **58**, 155.

6 Rockley, G. J. (1965). *Brit. med. J.*, **2**, 632.

7 Mykyta, L. J. (1968). *Med. J. Aust.*, **2**, 118.

CHAPTER 15

DRUGS WITH MAIN EFFECT ON AUTONOMIC NERVOUS SYSTEM

Amphetamines

Many doctors still persist in the unwarranted prescribing of amphetamines as appetite suppressants. In addition, they are given in the treatment of narcolepsy, mild depression, or parkinsonism. They are drugs of dependence and tolerance also occurs readily; this may be developed to a striking degree, especially in addicts. The stimulant and euphoriant effects are well-known, and these drugs are therefore frequently taken both orally and intravenously for 'kicks', specially by teenagers. If the dose is overestimated acute poisoning occurs and, regrettably, this is becoming more common.

The best known preparations are amphetamine sulphate (Benzedrine), dexamphetamine sulphate (Dexedrine) and methyl amphetamine (Methedrine).

The amphetamines are readily absorbed both from the gastrointestinal tract and from parenteral sites[1]. The metabolism has not been completely clarified but it is well established that approximately 50 per cent of an administered dose may be recovered in the urine as unchanged drug. The excretion is markedly pH dependent being considerably increased when the urine is acid; teenagers often take bicarbonate along with the amphetamine to prolong the effect of the drug.

The amphetamines are not inactivated by monoamine oxidase.

The toxic dose of amphetamine varies widely according to the degree of tolerance present. Blood levels are therefore of little value in assessing the severity of the poisoning.

Amphetamines may be measured in urine and blood. They may be very simply detected in urine by the methyl orange test.

Clinical Features

Assessment of the severity of poisoning must depend almost entirely on clinical signs.

CENTRAL NERVOUS SYSTEM. Alertness, talkativeness, restlessness, tremor, irritability and insomnia are commonly seen. Confusion, aggressiveness, anxiety, delirium, hallucinations, panic attacks and even suicidal or homicidal tendencies may occur. Increased limb reflexes are usual. The initial stimulant effect subsequently gives way to mental depression, lethargy and exhaustion. Convulsions and deep unconsciousness are characteristic of the terminal stages of very severe poisoning.

CARDIOVASCULAR SYSTEM. Headache, pallor, flushing, tachycardia, cardiac arrhythmias, angina pectoris, hypertension or hypotension. Circulatory collapse may occur.

GASTROINTESTINAL SYSTEM. Dryness of the mouth, anorexia, nausea, vomiting, diarrhoea and abdominal colic, which may be severe. Ulcers of the lips are common in addicts.

EFFECTS ON SKIN. Excessive sweating often occurs.

In fatal poisoning, the terminal stages are usually characterised by convulsions and deep unconsciousness.

For other features which may occur in addicts see page 185.

Treatment

The principles of therapy are described under Intensive Supportive Therapy (p. 18). Sedation is often indicated and is most successfully achieved with chlorpromazine[2], in children 1 mg per kg body weight intramuscularly and in adults 100 mg intramuscularly repeated at half-hourly intervals if necessary. If the amphetamine has been taken with a barbiturate, as is often the case, the chlorpromazine dosage should be halved.

There is inadequate information regarding the use of forced diuresis, peritoneal dialysis and haemodialysis, but as a considerable proportion of active drug is excreted in the urine forced acid diuresis is likely to be effective[3] (p. 35).

Fenfluramine

During the last 10 years this amphetamine derivative has come to be used widely in the treatment of obesity. In contrast to amphetamine, this compound in therapeutic dosage lacks central nervous stimulation[1] and has a low potential for inducing drug dependence[2]. Laboratory evidence supporting these conclusions includes an absence of influence of fenfluramine in therapeutic doses on critical flicker frequency[3] and R.E.M. sleep[4]. Acute overdosage has occurred in addicts who have used fenfluramine as a substitute for amphetamines and, because of its ready availability in many households, accidental and self-poisoning incidents are not uncommon. A number of fatalities have been recorded in children following heavy overdosage[5, 6], but in adults recovery has occurred following the acute ingestion of up to 90 tablets (20 mg).

Clinical Features

In acute overdosage the clinical features of fenfluramine toxicity are similar to those of amphetamines (p. 110). The most striking features are marked excitability and restlessness with sweating and hyperpyrexia. Fixed, dilated pupils, rotatory nystagmus and broxism are common[7]. Convulsions are likely in severe overdosage and, in reported cases, cardiac arrest is the usual mode of death.

Treatment

1. Gastric aspiration and lavage (p. 23).
2. Intensive supportive therapy (p. 18).
3. Forced acid diuresis has been advocated[7] although fenfluramine excretion is not markedly enhanced in the presence of acid urine[8].

Ephedrine

Ephedrine is prescribed as the sulphate or hydrochloride. It stimulates both α and β adrenergic receptors and owes part of its peripheral action to the release of noradrenaline. Like amphetamine, ephedrine is resistant to the action of monoamine oxidase.

Absorption occurs readily after oral administration or following subcutaneous and intramuscular injection. It is also effective topically in the form of nasal and eye drops. A high proportion of an administered dose is recovered unchanged in the urine.

Clinical Features

The signs and symptoms of ephedrine overdosage are similar to those of amphetamine poisoning. Features of paranoid psychosis, delusions and hallucinations may be prominent, but the other central nervous excitatory effects are less marked.

Treatment

Intensive supportive therapy (p. 18) should be given. Tachycardia and arrhythmias may be troublesome and rather resistant to treatment but a good response to adrenergic blocking drugs, such as practolol, is found. Practolol 100 mg should be given slowly intravenously, with full electrocardiographic control, followed by 100 mg twice daily orally, if required.

Isoprenaline (Isoproterenol)

This compound is presented as the hydrochloride, hydrogen tartrate and sulphate (Neo-Epinine). Isoprenaline is the most active of the sympathomimetic agents and exerts its pharmacological effect almost exclusively on β adrenergic receptors. It is readily absorbed when given parenterally or as an aerosol. The drug is also effective when given sublingually. Isoprenaline is rapidly detoxicated in the body by monoamine oxidase and by catechol-0-methyltransferase, and the metabolites so formed are excreted in the urine. Because of its rapid inactivation the effects of the drug are of short duration. In large overdosage, however, considerable amounts of isoprenaline itself may appear in the urine.

Clinical Features

The acute toxicity of isoprenaline is low. However, cardiac arrhythmias frequently occur, together with palpitations, tachycardia and headache. Anginal pain sometimes occurs even in subjects with no known myocardial disease. Nausea, tremor, dizziness and fatigue are also features of poisoning, and flushing of the skin may be evident.

Treatment

The symptomatic treatment of intensive supportive therapy (p. 18) is all that is necessary. In view of its predominantly β adrenergic effects, cardiac arrhythmias due to isoprenaline overdosage are most likely to respond to practolol administration.

The Belladonna Alkaloids

This group of compounds acts by inhibiting the muscarine effects of acetylcholine and so blocks the action of structures innervated by post-ganglionic cholinergic nerves and they also inhibit the response of smooth muscle to acetylcholine. Certain members of the group, including atropine in high dosage, block transmission at autonomic ganglia and skeletal neuromuscular junctions. The ganglion blocking action is particularly marked with the quaternary ammonium compounds of this group.

The belladonna alkaloids are readily absorbed from the alimentary tract; from topical application to mucosal surfaces and also from parenteral sites. The quaternary ammonium compounds are less well absorbed. All of these drugs are rapidly detoxicated in the liver, but a proportion is excreted unchanged by the kidney, in the few hours after absorption.

ATROPINE, SCOPOLAMINE AND HOMATROPINE

In adults, acute poisoning with these drugs is uncommon but they may be dangerous to children even in relatively small doses. Acute toxic effects may occur after apparently therapeutic doses given by eye instillation or by oral medication, as in the treatment of enuresis. Acute poisoning may also occur after ingesting various fruits or berries (p. 181) many of which contain belladonna alkaloids. The assessment of the severity of poisoning must be based on the clinical findings as there is a wide variation of response to these drugs.

Clinical Features

CENTRAL NERVOUS SYSTEM. Fixed dilated pupils. Blurring of vision and photophobia; ataxia; mental confusion, excitement, hallucinations and at times memory defect. These features are often so marked that they may lead to a mistaken diagnosis of acute psychiatric illness.

CARDIOVASCULAR SYSTEM. Tachycardia; hypertension; cardiac arrhythmias. In severe cases hypotension may develop and this is associated with a poor prognosis.

GASTROINTESTINAL SYSTEM. Dryness and burning of the mouth with marked thirst, abdominal distension with nausea and vomiting.

RENAL DISORDERS. Urinary urgency and possible acute retention.

METABOLIC DISORDER. Hyperpyrexia.

EFFECTS ON SKIN. Erythema and various skin rashes which may progress to exfoliation.

In severe intoxication the patient may enter a stage of central nervous depression with central failure of cardiovascular and respiratory function. Death, which is uncommon, except in children, usually results from respiratory failure.

Treatment

1. Intensive supportive therapy (p. 18) in a darkened room if photophobia is severe.

2. The peripheral effects may be alleviated by subcutaneous injection of carbachol (0·125 mg test dose, then if no untoward effect 0·5 mg) and neostigmine (0·25 mg). These drugs, however, do not influence the more dangerous central effects, particularly of atropine.
3. When central nervous stimulation is marked, sedation with a short acting barbiturate or diazepam may be necessary. A much more effective treatment for the central nervous effects is physostigmine salicylate which may be given intravenously, intramuscularly or subcutaneously depending on the severity of the situation. One to 4 mg of this drug will rapidly antagonise both the peripheral and central toxic effects of atropine. It should be recognised that physostigmine is rapidly metabolised and repeated doses may be required every 1-2 hours.
4. High pyrexia may be corrected by the use of a wet sheet and a fan.

PROPANTHELINE BROMIDE (PRO-BANTHINE)

This is the most commonly used quaternary ammonium derivative of the belladonna alkaloids. It has a potent ganglion blocking effect in addition to antimuscarine activity. The clinical features and treatment of acute overdosage are similar to atropine poisoning.

REFERENCES

Amphetamines
1 Innes, I. R. and Nickerson, M. (1970). Drugs acting on postganglionic adrenergic nerve endings and structures innervated by them (sympathomimetic drugs). In *The Pharmacological Basis of Therapeutics*, ed. Goodman, L. S. and Gilman, A., p. 501. New York: Collier.
2 Espelin, D. E. and Done, A. K. (1968). *New Engl. J. Med.*, **278**, 1361.
3 Zalis, E. G. and Parmley, L. F. (1963). *Arch. int. med.*, **112**, 822.

Fenfluramine
1 British Medical Association (1968). *Report of the Working Party on Amphetamine Preparations*.

116 TREATMENT OF COMMON ACUTE POISONINGS

2 Office of Health Economics (1969). *Obesity and Disease.* H.M.S.O.
3 Hill, R. C. and Turner, P. (1967). *J. Pharm. Pharmac.*, **19,** 337.
4 Oswald, I., Jones, H. S. and Mannerheim, J. E. (1968). *Brit. med. J.*, **1,** 796.
5 Fleisher, E. R. and Campbell, D. B. (1969). *Lancet*, **2,** 1306.
6 Campbell, D. B. and Moore, E. W. R. (1969). *Lancet*, **2,** 1307.
7 Riley, I., Corson, J., Haider, I. and Oswald, I. (1969). *Lancet*, **2,** 1162.
8 Beckett, A. H. and Brookes, L. G. (1967). *J. Pharm. Pharmac.*, **19,** Suppl., 425.

CHAPTER 16

ACUTE METALLIC POISONINGS

Iron Salts

There are a multitude of different therapeutic preparations of iron on the market, most of which are for oral administration. Many of these are put up in highly coloured tablets which are often available, in quantity, in homes with young families. Acute iron poisoning in children is therefore common and is an important cause of death in the younger age groups. Overdosage also occurs, not infrequently, in teenagers and adults. All preparations of iron are dangerous but some, such as ferrous gluconate, are considered rather less toxic.

Iron preparations are readily absorbed from the gastro-intestinal tract. Dilute solutions are mildly astringent, but when the concentration is high, as in acute overdosage, such solutions have marked corrosive properties. Damage to the gastric mucosa, therefore, may be severe. Necrosis and perforation of the stomach and bowel may occur and subsequent stricture formation is not infrequent.

The excretion of iron is normally very limited and most of an excess is ultimately taken up as apoferritin by the reticulo-endothelial system. A considerable improvement in the management of acute iron poisoning has resulted from the introduction of desferrioxamine, a potent iron chelating agent[1, 2], which both greatly restricts its absorption[3] and enhances its excretion.

The diagnosis of this poisoning may be confirmed by measuring iron levels in the plasma and gastric aspirate.

Clinical Features

The features are more severe in young children but this poisoning is potentially dangerous in all age groups. Acute iron poisoning occurs in three stages.

STAGE 1. After ingestion of the overdose, symptoms may appear either very rapidly or not for several hours. The predominant initial features are those of acute gastric disturbance, with epigastric pain, nausea and vomiting. Haematemesis is frequently evident but the vomit may be black in colour, due to the presence of iron in solution. The patient is usually pale or sometimes a curious grey colour. If gastrointestinal haemorrhage is severe, a state of shock will develop. Respiration and pulse are usually rapid.

STAGE 2. An interval of hours to even several days may elapse during which there are no further signs and symptoms. This may give rise to a mistaken impression that all is well, until frequent black and offensive stools are passed. Signs of acute encephalopathy may then appear, including severe headache, confusion, delirium, convulsions and loss of consciousness. Respiration becomes deep and rapid, and circulatory collapse may occur.

STAGE 3. In severe acute overdosage, death usually occurs in stage 2, but even if the patient survives this crisis recovery cannot be assured. Acute liver necrosis may develop, as evidenced by the appearance of jaundice; this sometimes progresses to hepatic coma and death. If jaundice is noted full assessment of liver function must be made. Oliguria and even anuria may develop and carry a poor prognosis[2, 4, 5].

LABORATORY FINDINGS. A level above 500 μg per 100 ml in a toddler and above 800 μg per 100 ml in an adult within four hours of ingestion indicates severe poisoning.

Treatment

Iron poisoning is potentially so dangerous that treatment is a matter of urgency. Where there is a reasonable suspicion that an overdose has been taken, it is better to act swiftly rather than wait for chemical confirmation of a high plasma iron level.

The basic principles of symptomatic treatment must be followed, according to intensive supportive therapy (p. 18).

In addition the following procedure should be undertaken.

1. *Gastric Aspiration and Lavage.* This should always be performed except when the patient is severely shocked. Lavage should be carried out using appropriate volumes of a solution of desferrioxamine (2 g) in 1 litre of warm water. Following lavage 10 g of desferrioxamine dissolved in 50 ml of water should be left in the stomach. This substance is not absorbed, but will chelate any free iron in the stomach and intestine. The chelate ferrioxamine is also poorly absorbed and, therefore, iron absorption is effectively blocked[3].

2. *Parenteral Desferrioxamine.* Immediately inject desferrioxamine (2 g in 10 ml water in an adult and 1 g in 5 ml water in a child) intramuscularly. In addition an intravenous drip should be set up, so that desferrioxamine may be given by continuous infusion at a rate of no more than 15 mg/kg per hour. The maximum dose by this route is 80 mg/kg per 24 hours. The intramuscular injection of 2 g of desferrioxamine should be repeated at 12-hourly intervals, according to the clinical state and plasma iron levels. This treatment depends on an adequate urinary flow, otherwise the chelate ferrioxamine is not excreted and may cause toxic effects in its own right[6]. If oliguria or anuria occur, therefore, haemodialysis or peritoneal dialysis must be started as a matter of urgency[5, 7].

Supplies of this iron chelating agent should be available for emergency use in every hospital casualty department.

Arsenic

Arsenic, the poison of melodrama, is seldom now encountered in clinical practice. Acute poisoning may arise from the ingestion of arsenic in weedkillers, rodenticides, insecticides or even medicines such as vaginal pessaries. In America arsenical pesticides cause more deaths in children than any other type of pesticide and of the heavy metals arsenic is the second commonest cause of death. Organic arsenicals are very much less likely to cause poisoning than inorganic derivatives. The acute toxic dose of trivalent inorganic salt is about 100 mg.

The chief toxic effects are on the alimentary system and they usually become apparent within one hour of ingestion but may be delayed for up to 12 hours.

Clinical Features

ALIMENTARY SYSTEM. Constriction in mouth and throat. Severe gastroenteritis, with copious watery stools which may contain blood; jaundice may appear after two days.

CARDIOVASCULAR SYSTEM. Tachycardia, hypotension, circulatory collapse.

RENAL DISORDERS. Oliguria or anuria. Urine contains albumen, blood and casts.

CENTRAL NERVOUS SYSTEM. Headache, irritability, muscular weakness, convulsions, and coma.

BLOOD FINDINGS. Haemolysis may occur but is rare.

METABOLIC DISORDER. Severe fluid and electrolyte imbalance may occur resulting in marked muscle cramps.

Treatment

It is important that the clinical diagnosis is confirmed by the detection of arsenic in the vomitus or stool before starting treatment, as this in itself can be dangerous.

1. Intensive supportive therapy (p. 18).
2. Treatment with dimercaprol should be initiated at once, without waiting for evidence of renal involvement; 4 mg/kg intramuscularly every four hours for 48 hours, followed by 3 mg/kg twice daily for eight days constitutes the maximum recommended dosage. These injections are painful and locally irritant. They should therefore be given in different sites successively.
3. Correction of dehydration may require copious intravenous fluids together with conventional measures to correct electrolyte imbalance.
4. Renal damage may be severe and require peritoneal dialysis (p. 36) or haemodialysis.
5. Liver damage may require conventional therapy, and where this fails exchange blood transfusion.

Gold

Gold has been used as a therapeutic agent for centuries but since 1930 it has come to be used widely in the treatment of arthritis. Acute poisoning, therefore, may result from injudicious or poorly controlled administration of gold. Toxicity is particularly liable if corticosteroid drugs are being given at the same time. Also toxic effects are found more commonly in older patients.

Clinical Features

DERMATOLOGICAL. The commonest effects are on skin and mucous membranes, usually the mouth. The changes in the skin range from erythema to exfoliative dermatitis often preceded by pruritis. Stomatitis, pharyngitis, tracheitis, gastritis, colitis and vaginitis all may occur.

HAEMATOLOGICAL. Severe blood dyscrasias may occur. Thrombocytopenia may be marked and is the usual cause of death. Leukopenia, agranulocytosis and aplastic anaemia are all liable. When major marrow depression occurs urinary coproporphyrin and delta-aminolaevulinic acid may increase markedly.

RENAL DISORDER. Albuminuria and haematuria and severe renal failure may result.

NEUROLOGICAL DISORDER. Encephalitis and peripheral neuritis are uncommon complications.

ALIMENTARY DISORDER. Nausea, vomiting and jaundice due to liver damage are occasionally found.

Treatment

If the symptoms are mild all that may be required is the withdrawal of the gold therapy. In more severe cases:—
1. Intensive supportive therapy (p. 18).
2. Dimercaprol (BAL) should be given as for arsenic poisoning (p. 120). In the unusual situation of adverse reaction to dimercaprol, penicillamine (250 mg capsules) 1-4 g orally daily is a suitable alternative.

3. Thrombocytopenia may require large doses of corticosteroid treatment. Other haematological problems may require vigorous treatment such as blood transfusion.

4. Renal failure should be treated by medical measures but if these fail peritoneal dialysis (p. 36) or haemodialysis may be required.

Mercury

Acute mercurial poisoning is commonly caused by oral ingestion of mercuric chloride or mercuric cyanide, although it may also result from inhalation of vapours of elemental mercury, organic mercurials or even by skin absorption of mercury containing ointments. It may also be encountered unexpectedly following the ingestion of other illegally manufactured preparations such as amphetamines which contain mercury contaminants. Mercury in its metallic form is not toxic when taken orally as it is not absorbed. The hazard from swallowing parts of a broken thermometer is that of the glass and not the mercury[1, 2]. Metallic mercury poisoning may, however, arise from the use of the metal as a seal in syringes for withdrawing specimens for blood gas analysis. Accidents may occur through faulty technique allowing metallic mercury to enter the circulation[3].

Mercurous chloride (Calomel) and the organic mercurial preparations which are used as fungicides, are unlikely to cause serious acute toxic effects, even in large doses, as they are so poorly absorbed.

Mercuric chloride (corrosive sublimate) is used as a strong disinfectant and is highly toxic; the fatal dose can be as little as 0·5 g. The chief effect is on the kidney.

Clinical Features

ALIMENTARY SYSTEM. Grey appearance and pain of mouth or pharynx. Nausea, vomiting, thirst and severe colic with bloody stools. Metallic taste. Jaundice may develop later.

CARDIOVASCULAR SYSTEM. Tachycardia, hypotension and shock.

RENAL DISORDERS. Oliguria or anuria develop within 48 hours of ingestion. The urine contains much albumen, and some blood and casts.

RESPIRATORY SYSTEM. If the poisoning is by inhalation pneumonitis may result with associated tachypnoea and cyanosis.

CENTRAL NERVOUS SYSTEM. Lethargy, excitement, hyper-reflexia and tremor.

METABOLIC DISORDER. Dehydration and electrolyte upset may be severe.

The systemic features usually start within a few hours and may last for several days.

Treatment

1. Intensive supportive therapy (p. 18). In poisoning by ingestion gastric lavage should be done if possible using 250 ml of 5 per cent solution of sodium formaldehyde sulphoxylate and then a further 100 ml should be left in the stomach after lavage. This substance reduces bivalent mercuric ion to the much less soluble mercurous form and so the absorption of the mercury is reduced.
2. Dimercaprol (BAL) should be given at once, as for arsenic poisoning (p. 120).
3. Oliguria or anuria should be treated by routine medical measures initially but if these fail peritoneal dialysis (p. 36) or haemodialysis may be necessary.
4. In the unlikely event of an adverse reaction to dimercaprol, penicillamine should be tried. The place, however, of this remedy in the treatment of acute mercury poisoning has not yet been fully evaluated.

Lead

Although chronic lead poisoning is being recognised with increasing frequency, acute lead poisoning arises very seldom. Acute toxic effects due to lead result from ingestion of soluble or rapidly absorbed compounds of lead. Acute plumbism may also occur in the course of chronic poisoning as a result of intercurrent illness or change in acid-base state for any reason, but especially during treatment of chronic lead intoxication. Although, as a result of stringent industrial controls, acute poisoning with organic lead substances, such as tetraethyl and tetramethyl lead, is very uncommon, the slightest indiscretion in handling these compounds is likely to result in acute toxic effects. Not only are they volatile and so may be inhaled but they are markedly fat soluble and may be absorbed on contact with the skin.

Acute lead poisoning is almost always accidental in workers exposed to this hazard, but may occur also in children as a result of sucking or eating lead containing materials such as certain paints.

Clinical Features

The main effects tend to be on the alimentary system.

ALIMENTARY SYSTEM. Marked thirst and metallic taste; nausea and vomiting, the vomitus often being white in colour due to the formation of lead chloride; colic which may be very severe; diarrhoea, the stool usually being black due to the presence of lead disulphide.

CENTRAL NERVOUS SYSTEM. Parasthesiae, muscle pain and fatigue; convulsions and loss of consciousness.

CARDIOVASCULAR SYSTEM. Hypotension and circulatory collapse.

BLOOD FINDINGS. Severe anemia due to an acute haemolytic crisis may occur.

RENAL DISORDERS. Oliguria or anuria may result.

HEPATIC DISORDER. Acute liver failure is an occasional complication.

LABORATORY FINDINGS. Porphyrinuria, mainly due to coproporphyrin III, although not diagnostic, is a valuable screening test for lead poisoning. More definitive investigations are measurements of levels of lead in the blood and urine. In the blood, levels above 0·07 mg per 100 ml are indicative of acute intoxication. Levels above this are approximately proportional to the severity of the poisoning, but if above 1·0 mg per 100 ml the test should be repeated as contamination of the specimen has almost certainly occurred. In the urine an output of lead of 0·15-0·30 mg per litre measured on 24 hour collections of urine is in keeping with acute lead poisoning.

Treatment

1. Gastric aspiration and lavage (p. 23) is important in patients who have recently ingested lead.

2. Intensive supportive therapy (p. 18).

3. If acute encephalopathy predominates cerebral oedema is marked and the patient will be made worse if intravenous fluids are given. In these cases, for the first 24 hours the chelating agents should be given intramuscularly in the dosage given below and cautious mannitol infusion (p. 60) should be added to the regimen to reduce intracranial pressure.

4. The combination of British Anti-Lewisite (BAL) and calcium disodium versenate (Versene-Riker) has been shown to be much more effective than if the versenate is used alone. This combination will achieve a sufficient molar excess of chelating agent over lead. The dosage schedule is calcium disodium versenate 75 mg/kg body weight intravenously in 24 hours plus BAL 24 mg/kg intramuscularly in 24 hours. This regimen should be continued for three to five days.

5. If there is significant renal impairment the above regimen must be combined with peritoneal or haemodialysis.

6. Where colic is severe calcium gluconate (10 per cent) 10 ml intravenously may provide relief, but in some patients pethidine or morphine may be required. Time should not be wasted in attempts to evacuate residual lead from the bowel by enemata.

7. Convulsions should be controlled by diazepam 10 mg intravenously supplemented if necessary by sodium phenobarbitone 200 mg intramuscularly.

8. During convalescence long term control of plumbism will be achieved by the oral administration of d-penicillamine 20-40 mg/kg daily.

Phosphorus

Phosphorous may be encountered in two distinct forms, the red granular which is not poisonous and the highly toxic, yellow, waxy, fat soluble and water insoluble form. Yellow phosphorus is used in fireworks and matches (p. 161) and in rodent and insect poisons. Poisoning is usually by ingestion but skin and lungs may be the source of entry.

Clinical Features

The main toxic effects are on the liver leading to acute hepatic failure.

GATROINTESTINAL SYSTEM. Nausea, vomiting and profuse diarrhoea.

HEPATIC DISORDERS. Liver enlarged and tender; jaundice and acute liver failure. Hypoprothrombinaemia.

CARDIOVASCULAR SYSTEM. Hypotension and 'shock'.

METABOLIC DISORDER. Acidosis may be marked.

RENAL DISORDERS. Oliguria and anuria. The urine may contain red cells.

CENTRAL NERVOUS SYSTEM. Delirium and coma. These are usually terminal features in fatal cases.

Treatment

1. Gastric aspiration and lavage (p. 23) using 0·1 per cent copper sulphate in water.
2. Intensive supportive therapy (p. 18).
3. Vitamin K_1, 20 mg intravenously and repeated according to the prothrombin time.
4. In severe liver failure apart from the routine medical measures of diet, etc., hydrocortisone 100 mg intravenously four times daily is of benefit. When routine measures fail exchange blood transfusion should be considered.

5. If renal failure is severe peritoneal or haemodialysis may be required.
6. Phosphorus burns should be thoroughly washed with 1 per cent copper sulphate solution in water.

REFERENCES

Iron

1 Westlin, W. F. (1966). *Clin. Pediatrics*, **5**, 531.
2 Barr, D. G. D. and Fraser, D. K. B. (1968). *Brit. med. J.*, **1**, 737.
3 Wohler, F. (1964). In *Iron Metabolism*, ed. Gross, F., Naegeli, S. R. and Philips, H. D., p. 561 *et sqq*. Berlin: Springer Verlag.
4 Drysdale, A. E. and Powell, L. W. (1964). *Med. J. Aust.*, **2**, 990.
5 Lavender, S. and Bell, J. A. (1970). *Brit. med. J.*, **2**, 406.
6 Whitten, C. F., You-Chen Chen and Gibson, G. W. (1966). *Pediatrics*, **38**, 102.
7 Covey, T. J. (1964). *J. Pediatrics*, **64**, 218.

Mercury

1 Mofenson, H. and Greensher, J. (1973). *J. Am. med. Ass.*, **223**, 559.
2 Johnson, H. R. M. and Koumides, O. (1967). *Brit. med. J.*, **1**, 340.
3 Cook, T. A. and Yates, P. O. (1969). *Brit. Dental J.*, **2**, 553.

Lead

1 Barltrop, D. (1969). *Brit. J. Hospital Med.*, **2** (9), 1567
2 Guinee, V. F. (1972). *Am. J. Med.*, **52** (3), 283.
3 *Clinical Toxicology Bulletin* (1973). Vol. **3**, Nos. 2 and 3.

CHAPTER 17

THE ALCOHOLS

Methyl Alcohol (Methanol)

Methyl alcohol (wood alcohol) can produce serious poisoning, both by inhalation and ingestion. A common source of this poisoning is the taking of methylated spirits but it is also contained in certain home made beverages, anti-freeze, paint removers and varnish[1, 2]. It is much more toxic than ethyl alcohol, probably because it is metabolised to formic acid or formaldehyde, both of which severely inhibit essential metabolic processes[3]. The enzymic oxidation of methanol proceeds at one-fifth of the rate of the corresponding reaction with ethanol. Hence in the treatment of poisoning by methanol, the administration of ethanol slows the rate of accumulation of toxic products[4].

Clinical Features

Since methanol is distributed in the tissues according to their water content, a high concentration is found in the vitreous body and optic nerve and the consequent impairment of vision is a characteristic feature of the poisoning. As one of the principle metabolites is formic acid severe metabolic acidosis occurs.

Headache, nausea and vomiting. Severe abdominal pain.

Blurring of vision, which may lead to blindness.

Dilation of pupils and papilloedema.

Acidotic breathing.

Initial restlessness followed by loss of consciousness of varying degree.

Laboratory findings of severe metabolic acidosis.

Blood level of above 300 mg per 100 ml indicates severe poisoning.

Treatment

1. Gastric aspiration and lavage if discovered within four hours (p. 23).
2. The acidosis must be treated energetically with appropriate intravenous infusions of sodium bicarbonate.
3. Ethyl alcohol 50 per cent, 1 ml/kg should be given orally at once followed by 0·5 ml/kg every two hours for five days.
4. If there is impaired vision and the response to these measures is unsatisfactory, haemodialysis (p. 41) or peritoneal dialysis (p. 36) is essential. Haemodialysis is the method of choice since it will reduce the blood levels of formic acid and formaldehyde more rapidly.

The metabolism of methanol is slow and there is, therefore, a considerable risk of recurrence of the toxic features even after a successful period of treatment. The patient should be kept under close observation for several days before recovery is considered complete.

Ethyl Alcohol

This is a frequent cause of acute poisoning by its production of inebriation. It is widely used in industry and elsewhere and may be taken by accident, when stored in incorrectly labelled bottles. Ethyl alcohol is frequently taken in addition to other drugs in the course of self-poisoning and this may occur in up to 70 per cent of these incidents.

The fatal dose is difficult to ascertain because of individual tolerance (the result of habituation) but the equivalent of about 400 ml of pure ethyl alcohol consumed in one hour may be lethal.

Ethyl alcohol is rapidly absorbed from the upper gastro-intestinal tract and is distributed in the tissues according to their water content, like methyl alcohol[5, 6]. The main effect is that of a central nervous depressant.

Clinical Features

Inebriation.

Muscular incoordination. Blurred vision.

Impaired reaction time.

Excitement due to loss of inhibitions.

Impairment of consciousness. Coma.

Tachycardia. Slow respiration.

A blood alcohol of 80 mg per 100 ml will produce recognisable features of drunkenness. A level above 300 mg per 100 ml is dangerous to life. A high degree of tolerance may develop in people habituated to ethyl alcohol, however, and clinical assessment of this poisoning is therefore essential.

In children severe hypoglycaemia and convulsions may occur.

Treatment

1. Gastric aspiration and lavage (p. 23) are important.
2. Intensive supportive therapy (p. 18).
3. In very severe poisoning peritoneal dialysis or haemodialysis[7] may be necessary.
4. Intravenous infusion of 200 g of fructose (500 ml of a 40 per cent solution) over a 30 minute period is of value as it has been shown to increase the rate of fall of blood ethanol by about 25 per cent[8]. This may cause symptoms of retrosternal and epigastric discomfort and, more important, acidaemia which should be corrected by the administration of alkali if it occurs.

Delirium Tremens

It is now generally accepted that this is a true withdrawal state although thiamine and nicotinic acid deficiencies may be added factors. It usually occurs in a chronic alcoholic following a drinking bout.

Clinical Features

Hallucinations, usually visual and inducing intense fear.

Sleeplessness, restlessness, agitation and delirium. Profuse sweating is common. Grand mal convulsions may occur. Tachycardia. Hypotension. Clover-shaped S-T changes are evident in the electrocardiagram; these are often said to be diagnostic of chronic alcoholism.

Treatment

1. Chlorpromazine (100 mg intramuscularly) and repeat thereafter as required with due regard for the development of hypotension[8]. Sodium amytal (200 mg.) may profitably be combined with the doses of chlorpromazine. Several controlled studies [9, 10] have demonstrated that paraldehyde and chlordiazepoxide are superior to phenothiazines in the treatment of delirium tremens and that their use significantly reduces the mortality. Heminevrin has also been advocated, but in our experience the combined treatment with chlorpromazine and sodium amytal has proved most effective.
2. Parentrovite Forte, 40 ml intravenously on the few occasions when there are any associated features of Korsakoff's psychosis or Wernicke's encephalopathy.
4. Fluid and electrolyte balance maintained by intravenous infusion of 500 ml. N. Saline and 1,000 ml 5 per cent dextrose in rotation. These patients are often considerably dehydrated and may require 6·0 litres to correct this. Hypomagnesaemia may be marked and so the plasma magnesium level should always be measured and corrected as required by appropriate administration of supplements.

Prognosis

Delirium tremens is a serious medical emergency and requires expert supervision if a fatal outcome is to be avoided. Infection is common, both as a precipitant and a complication of delirium tremens, and must be treated energetically.

Disulfiram (Antabuse)

The ingestion of disulfiram itself in toxic amounts will give rise to psychotic behaviour and central nervous system depression, for which symptomatic treatment is adequate[11]. The drug is used in the treatment of alcoholics and is intended to give rise to an adverse reaction if ethyl alcohol is taken. Disulfiram interferes with the metabolism of ethyl alcohol and the resulting toxic effects are due to the accumulation of acetaldehyde. As disulfiram is excreted very slowly such effects may occur for at least three weeks following the last ingestion of the drug.

The formation of acetaldehyde results in toxic effects mainly on the cardiovascular system.

Clinical Features

CARDIOVASCULAR SYSTEM. Tachycardia, arryhthmias and hypotension which may be severe. Cardiac failure.

CENTRAL NERVOUS SYSTEM. Agitation, progressing to drowsiness. Convulsions may occur.

GASTROINTESTINAL SYSTEM. Nausea and vomiting.

METABOLIC DISORDERS. Flushing, sweating and tachypnoea—due to acidosis.

LABORATORY FINDINGS. Blood alcohol levels above 50 mg per 100 ml are dangerous when disulfiram has also been taken.

Treatment

1. Intensive supportive therapy (p. 18).
2. Vitamin C (ascorbic acid) 500 mg intravenously and repeated in one hour.
3. In very severe reactions treatment as for ethyl alcohol poisoning (p. 130).

REFERENCES

1 Murdoch Ritchie, J. (1970). The Aliphatic Alcohols. In *The Pharmacological Basis of Therapeutics*, ed. Goodman, L. S. and Gilman, A., p. 145. New York: Collier.

2 Cooper, J. R. and Kini, M. M. (1962). *Biochem. Pharmac.*, **11,** 405.

3 Mardones, J. (1963). The Alcohols. In *Physiological Pharmacology*, Vol. 1, ed. Root, W. S. and Hofmann, F. G. New York: Academic Press.

4   Smith, M. E. (1961).   *J. Pharmac. exp. Ther.*, **134,** 233.
5   Forney, R. B. and Harger, R. N. (1969).   *Ann. Rev. Pharmacol.*, **9,** 379.
6   Wallgren, H. and Barry, H. (1970).   *Actions of Alcohol, Vol.* 1, p. 100.   Amsterdam: Elsevier.
7   Leader (1969).   *Scot. med. J.*, **14,** 263.
8   Brown, S. S., Forrest, J. A. H. and Roscoe, P. (1972).   *Lancet*, **2,** 898.
9   Golbert, T. M., Sanz, C. J., Rose, H. D. and Leitschuh, T. H. (1967). *J. Am. med. Ass.*, **201,** 99.
10 Kaim, S. C., Klett, C. J. and Rothfield, B. (1969).   *Amer. J. Psychiat.*, **25,** 1640.
11 Victor, M. (1966).   *Psychosom. Med.*, **28,** 636.

CHAPTER 18

DIGITALIS, QUININE AND QUINIDINE

Digitalis

Preparations of digitalis are available in many households and may be taken for self-poisoning by adults or accidentally by children[1]. The fatal dose in an adult for most preparations is about 30 times the daily maintenance dose. It is important, however, to be aware that despite few symptoms and only minor ECG changes such as first degree A-V block, sudden deterioration in the cardiac state may occur. The degree of block may become severe or myocardial excitability rapidly increase. The likely cause of this deterioration is myocardial depletion of potassium, evidenced by a rise in plasma potassium. This is probably due to inhibition of the membrane ATP-ase pump and may be corrected rapidly by intravenous glucose and soluble insulin. Plasma potassium levels, determined 3-18 hours after ingestion of a toxic amount of digitalis, are a more helpful prognostic guide than the initial ECG[2, 3].

Clinical Features

Nausea, vomiting and diarrhoea are commonly found.

Bradycardia, which may be severe.

Varying degrees of atrioventricular block. Ectopic beats, particularly ventricular ectopic beats; coupled rhythm; ventricular tachycardia and ventricular fibrillation. These arrhythmias may be complex and electrocardiographic monitoring is essential.

Drowsiness, mental confusion and even psychosis may occur.

Hyper- or hypokalaemia.

Raised plasma digoxin levels which do not correlate, however, with the severity of poisoning.

Treatment
1. Intensive supportive therapy (p. 18). Gastric aspiration and lavage, if indicated (p. 23), should be undertaken with care as any increase in vagal tone may predispose to cardiac arrest.
2. Bradycardia should be treated with atropine sulphate, 0·6 mg intravenously, repeated as necessary, often for as long as four days.
3. Hyperkalaemia should be corrected by intravenous infusion of 50 g glucose and 20 units soluble insulin intramuscularly.
4. Hypokalaemia should be treated by cautious intravenous infusion of 1 g potassium chloride in 200 ml 5 per cent dextrose. This should be continued until either the ECG or the plasma potassium level is normal.
5. Lignocaine 100 mg intravenously as a bolus followed by lignocaine 500 mg in 500 ml saline given at an infusion rate depending on the clinical response and the absence of hypotension, is now the most effective treatment for ventricular ectopic beats. If ventricular fibrillation occurs external cardiac massage and electrical defibrillation are necessary.
6. A high urine output should be maintained using mannitol diuresis (p. 35). This is not always possible in view of shock but this should improve rapidly by correction of the associated electrolyte disturbance or dysrhythmia.
7. There can be no doubt that a cardiac demand pacemaker in the right ventricle is highly desirable in the light of the possible sudden deterioration already mentioned[4].

Careful biochemical control is essential during the course of treatment.

Quinine and Quinidine

Quinine and quinidine are chemically optical isomers. Quinine has been mainly used as an antimalarial; it is also a constituent of many so-called 'tonics' and is often prescribed to prevent night cramps. It also has an ill-deserved reputation as an abortifacient and may be taken in deliberate overdosage in order to produce what is thought will be a really effective abortion. Quinidine, which is a potent cardiac depressant, is used in the treatment of cardiac arrhythmias. Both substances are taken occasionally in episodes of self-poisoning and may also be swallowed accidentally by children.

Clinical Features

Absorption is rapid but fortunately is considerably lessened by the almost inevitable vomiting which these drugs cause.

Both drugs may cause cinchonism; singing in the ears, deafness, blurred vision, headache and dizziness soon occur. Collapse with impairment of consciousness, shallow, rapid breathing, fast pulse with low blood pressure may follow. Cardiac arrhythmias and arrest may occur. Electrocardiographic changes include widening of the QRS complex and flattening of T waves.

Blurring of vision, dilated pupils or annular scotoma, and deafness, may persist for several days whilst in rare instances blindness may be permanent. Retinal examination may reveal marked constriction of the retinal vessels, the appearances resembling occlusion of the central retinal artery. Debate continues as to the mechanism of the visual loss. It is thought to be due either to a direct toxic effect on the ganglion cells of the retina or to quinine producing vasoconstriction and consequent retinal damage. The rapid response to stellate ganglion block mentioned below strongly supports the latter view[1].

Acute intravascular haemolysis may occur, the first warning of which may be diminished renal output.

Treatment

1. Intensive supportive therapy (p. 18).
2. Very careful observation of the heart rate and rhythm is essential, preferably by cardiac monitoring. Any arrhythmias must be treated with appropriate drugs such as propranolol or intravenous lignocaine.

3. Stellate ganglion block may produce dramatic relief of the visual impairment. The degree of visual improvement is inversely proportional to the duration of the blindness. Unfortunately these measures are not very effective but should be tried when there is severe impairment of vision.

4. Acute haemolysis requires treatment with intravenous hydrocortisone together with treatment of any associated acute renal failure.

5. Because both quinine and quinidine are largely protein bound, peritoneal dialysis and haemodialysis are not likely to recover a significant amount of these drugs[2]. Quinine and its congeners are largely metabolised in the liver so that less than 5 per cent of an administered dose appears unaltered in the urine. The amount recovered in the urine is doubled if the urine is made acid, and so in very severe poisoning forced diuresis with ammonium chloride (p. 35) to produce an acid urine may be of some value.

REFERENCES

Digitalis

1 Leader (1972). *Scot. med. J.*, **17**, 263.

2 Citrin, D., Stevenson, I. H. and O'Malley, K. (1972). *Scot. med. J.*, **17**, 275.

3 Bismuth, C., Gaultier, M., Conso, F. and Efthymiou, M. L. (1973). *Clin. Toxicol.* **6** (2), 153).

4 Cirtin, D. L., O'Malley, K. and Hillis, W. S. (1973). *Brit. med. J.*, **2**, 526.

Quinine

1 Bankes, J. L. K., Hayward, J. A. and Jones, M. B. S. (1972). *Brit. med. J.*, **4**, 85.

2 Donadio, J. V., Whelton, A., Gilliland, P. F. and Cirksena, W. J. (1968). *J. Am. med. Ass.*, **204**, 274.

CHAPTER 19

OPIUM ALKALOIDS AND MORPHINE DERIVATIVES

This is a large group and includes morphine, heroin, methadone, pethidine, codeine, dihydrocodeine, pentazocine, propoxyphene, diphenoxylate and dipipanone amongst many other potent analgesics. Acute poisoning may occur in a variety of ways. They are drugs of addiction (p. 184) and so are often in the possession of individuals who are prone to engage in self-poisoning. Accidental poisoning, particularly with the more potent drugs of this group, for example morphine and heroin, may be seen in addicts who, on admission to hospital, because of their lack of skill in intravenous injection, overestimate their dose requirements. On injection of the stated dose by an expert, frank poisoning may ensue. Acute toxic effects may also result from the injudicious administration of morphine to a patient with respiratory failure.

Fortunately acute poisoning with the potent members of this group of drugs is uncommon, but acute overdosage of codeine which is contained in many readily available proprietary mixtures of 'APC' (aspirin, phenacetin and codeine) is frequently found. The main features of these are usually due to the aspirin in the mixture (p. 69), but codeine may also be a significant factor.

The clinical features of poisoning due to these drugs may be described under the one heading, but the severity of the effects depends on the potency of the preparation taken.

Tolerance, particularly in addicts may be present to a high degree and so assessment of the severity of the overdosage largely depends on the clinical response of the patient.

Clinical Features

CENTRAL NERVOUS SYSTEM. Impaired level of consciousness which may be severe. The presence of pin-point pupils is a marked feature. Convulsions may occur particularly in young children. The skeletal muscles are usually flaccid but muscle twitching occurs especially in acute cocaine poisoning.

RESPIRATORY SYSTEM. Depression of respiration is usually a prominent effect.

CARDIOVASCULAR SYSTEM. Hypotension.

METABOLIC DISORDER. Hypothermia may occur.

HAEMATOLOGICAL FINDING. Methaemoglobinaemia may occur in codeine overdose.

In fatal poisonings death is usually due to respiratory depression.

Treatment

This is one of the very few occasions when a true antidote, a specific pharmacological antagonist is available. Nalorphine and levallorphan have been used routinely as specific antagonists for narcotic overdosage. These compounds are not ideal antagonists as they also have agonist actions and may provoke cardiovascular and severe respiratory depression[1, 2]. Also they are ineffective in reversing the effects of pentazocine[2].

Naloxone (N-allylnoroxymorphone) has in recent years been advocated as the antagonist of choice for the treatment of narcotic overdosage as it does not cause respiratory or cardiovascular depression, psychotogenic actions or drug dependence [2, 3]. It is also the only effective antagonist in the management of pentazocine poisoning. Naloxone acts very rapidly and the dramatic improvement in the patient is usually maintained although relapse may occur requiring repeated doses of naloxone. In view of its potency this antagonist should be used with caution in patients dependent on narcotics as it may precipitate acute withdrawal features.

1. Gastric aspiration and lavage (p. 23) if the drug has been ingested.
2. Intensive supportive therapy (p. 18).

3. Naloxone 0·4 mg intravenously and 0·8 mg repeated intravenously three minutes later, if necessary, is usually an adequate dose but larger doses may be required in heavy overdosage. Parenteral doses as high as 24 mg per 70 kg have been given without ill-effect.

If naloxone is not available, nalorphine hydrobromide (Lethidrone) should be given 15 mg intravenously every 15 minutes until consciousness is regained and respiration normal. Relapse may occur, in which event nalorphine in the above dose should be repeated. In very severe poisoning the initial dose, which, however, should not be repeated, can be 40 mg.

The patient must be closely observed after treatment with either naloxone or nalorphine as relapses may occur requiring repeated doses of these antagonists.

Prognosis

Provided naloxone and nalorphine are available and adequate doses are given, recovery from the acute overdosage can be confidently anticipated, but withdrawal features in an addict will require careful treatment.

Propoxyphene

Since its synthesis by Pohland and Sullivan in 1953[1], dextropropoxyphene hydrochloride has become a widely used analgesic. In Great Britain, for example, national health service prescriptions for this drug increased from 1,705,000 in 1968 to 2,500,000 in 1970. This trend continues and so acute poisoning is not uncommon.

Preparations are available either of dextropropoxyphene itself or more often in combination with another analgesic. These include:

Dextropropoxyphene Caps. B.P. containing 30 mg dextropropoxyphene HCl.

Darvon (Lilly) containing 32 mg dextropropoxyphene HCl.

Distalgesic (Dista) containing
$$\begin{cases} 32\cdot5 \text{ mg dextropropoxyphene} \\ \quad \text{HCl.} \\ 325 \text{ mg paracetamol.} \end{cases}$$

Doloxene (Lilly) containing 65 mg dextropropoxyphene HCl.

Doloxytal (Lilly) containing
$$\begin{cases} 65 \text{ mg dextropropoxyphene} \\ \quad \text{HCl.} \\ 30 \text{ mg amylobarbitone.} \end{cases}$$

Doloxene Compound-65
(Lilly) containing
$$\begin{cases} 65 \text{ mg dextropropoxyphene HCl.} \\ 162 \text{ mg phenacetin.} \\ 227 \text{ mg aspirin.} \\ 32\cdot4 \text{ mg caffeine.} \end{cases}$$

Depronal S.A. (Warner) containing 150 mg dextropropoxyphene HCl.

Dextropropoxyphene has a chemical structure related to methadone and produces analgesia by central action on the nervous system. When given orally it has approximately the same potency as an analgesic as codeine, and its side-effects also resemble codeine (p. 139) but there is less nausea and vomiting[2]. Dextropropoxyphene is rapidly absorbed from the gastrointestinal tract and it is then metabolised in the liver by demethylation and only about 10 per cent of an administered dose can be recovered unchanged in the urine after 24 hours[3]. The drug is poorly soluble in water but it is thought that it may have a high fat solubility and so large quantities may be stored rapidly in fat tissue[4]. This may explain why plasma levels of dextropropoxyphene remain very low (a few μg/ml) even in heavy overdosage. It may also explain the fluctuant course, which tends to occur in severely poisoned patients, as considerable quantities of drug may move out of fat stores some time after the patient's condition has apparently improved.

Problems of drug abuse and dependency with dextropropoxyphene were for many years thought to be insignificant and formal controls were not considered necessary[5, 6]. More recently, however, especially in the United States, drug abuse with dextropropoxyphene has become common in the armed forces and the population generally, and now the drug is severely proscribed in many major hospitals in North America.

Clinical Features

It should be noted that the patient's condition may fluctuate markedly during the first 24 hours and severe loss of consciousness, convulsions and respiratory and cardiac arrest may occur suddenly even when the patient is apparently recovering satisfactorily.

CENTRAL NERVOUS SYSTEM. Confusion, hallucinations, stammer, ataxia, vertigo and diplopia are common. Small or pin-point pupils. Convulsions may be followed rapidly by coma. In the recovery stage there may be marked sleep disturbance, particularly if the patient is habituated to the drug.

CARDIOVASCULAR SYSTEM. Tachycardia. Hypertension and hypotension. Cerebrovascular accidents and subarachnoid haemorrhage have been reported. Cardiac arrest, which is thought to occur mainly as a result of central brain damage rather than primary cardiac effect.

RESPIRATORY SYSTEM. Respiratory failure and arrest may occur.

GASTROINTESTINAL SYSTEM. Nausea and vomiting. Jaundice and other abnormal liver function tests may be found.

HAEMATOLOGICAL SYSTEM. Thrombocytopenia and macrocytic anaemia have been reported especially in patients chronically treated with the drug.

SKIN. Skin reactions may be very varied. Urticaria and pruritus are the most common.

Treatment

1. Gastric aspiration and lavage (p. 23).
2. Intensive supportive therapy as detailed (p. 18).
3. Nalorphine hydrobromide (Lethidrone) 15 mg intravenously every 15 minutes until consciousness is regained and respiration normal has been advocated, but the results in this poisoning have been variable[7, 8]. Naloxone 0·4-1·2 mg intravenously (p. 140) is more effective[9].

4. Convulsions may require strenuous treatment either by diazepam 10 mg intravenously or sodium phenobarbitone 200 mg intramuscularly.
5. Haemodialysis has been strongly recommended and its use has been suggested early in treatment in an effort to avoid the episodes of sudden deterioration which may occur[4].

The quantitative recovery of dextropropoxyphene is, however, low as would be expected with very low plasma levels and, therefore, the use of this treatment is of doubtful value. In any event the coma should be and is rapidly corrected by naloxone. There is, therefore, no indication for haemodialysis.

With the combined preparations of dextropropoxyphene the other drugs present may cause important toxic effects requiring specific treatment in their own right.

Diphenoxylate (Lomotil)

Lomotil (Searle) tablets contain 2·5 mg diphenoxylate hydrochloride and 0·025 mg atropine sulphate. This preparation is prescribed commonly for the treatment of diarrhoea even when this is relatively trivial and self-limiting. Diphenoxylate hydrochloride is chemically related to pethidine but its onset of action is slower and its duration more prolonged than other opiates. The dangers of acute overdosage, especially in young children, are not well recognised despite a number of recent reports stressing the toxicity of this poisoning[1-6].

Clinical Features

The toxic effects are influenced by the slow absorption, which is delayed further by the atropine action, and long duration of action of the drug. The patient may remain well, therefore, for many hours after ingestion and it may be several days before recovery is complete. Relapses are likely during the course of the poisoning.

RESPIRATORY SYSTEM. Respiratory depression is the main complication, especially in children, and may be severe. Apnoea due to depression of the respiratory centre may occur and is the major cause of death.

CARDIOVASCULAR SYSTEM. Hypotension and bradycardia also due to central depression. Cardiac arrest may occur.

CENTRAL NERVOUS SYSTEM. Impaired level of consciousness which may be severe. Pin-point pupils. Convulsions may develop, especially in young children.

METABOLIC DISORDER. Hypothermia may be severe.

Treatment

1. Intensive supportive therapy (p. 18).
2. Gastric aspiration and lavage (p. 23).
3. Naloxone 0·4 to 1·2 mg intravenously (p. 140) is an effective antagonist but repeated doses may be necessary in view of the duration of the toxic effects. If naloxone is not available, nalorphine hydrobromide (Lethidrone) 15 mg intravenously should be given and again repeated injections may be required every 15 minutes depending on the level of consciousness and the state of respiration. In toddlers the doses of nalorphine range from 0·25 mg to 2 mg intravenously.

Prognosis

Provided naloxone or nalorphine are available and administered in adequate doses the response to treatment should be satisfactory. It is very important, however, to monitor the patient's condition carefully for at least three days to ascertain that recovery is complete.

REFERENCES

Opium Alkaloids

1 Foldes, F. F., Duncalf, D., Kuwabara, S. (1969). *Can. Anaesth. Soc. J.*, **16**, 151.
2 Evans, L. E. J., Swainson, C. P., Roscoe, P., Prescott, L. F. (1973). *Lancet*, **1**, 452.
3 Jasinski, D. R., Martin, W. R., Haertzen, C. A. (1967). *J. Pharmac. exp. Ther.*, **157**, 420.

Propoxyphene

1 Pohland, A. and Sullivan, H. R. (1953). *J. Am. Chem. Soc.*, **75**, 4458.
2 Lasagna, L. (1964). *Pharmac. Rev.*, **16**, 47.
3 Way, E. L. and Adler, T. K. (1960). *Pharmac. Rev.*, **12**, 383.
4 Gary, N. E., Maher, J. F., De Myttenaere, M. H., Liggero, S. H., Scott, K. G., Matusiak, W. and Schreiner, G. E. (1968). *Arch. Int. Med.*, **121**, 453.
5 Fraser, H. F. and Isbell, H. (1960). *Bull. Narcot.*, **12**, 9.
6 Jaffe, J. H. (1967). In *The Pharmacological Basis of Therapeutics*, ed. Goodman, L. S. and Gilman, A., p. 279. New York: Collier.
7 Swarts, C. L. (1964). *Am. J. Dis. Child*, **63**, 158.
8 Karliner, J. S. (1967). *J. Am. Med. Ass.*, **199**, 1006.
9 Evans, L. E. J., Roscoe, P., Swainson, C. P. and Prescott, L. F. (1973). *Lancet*, **1**, 452.

Diphenoxylate

1 Harris, J. T. and Rossiter, M. (1969). *Lancet*, **1**, 150.
2 Henderson, W. and Psaila, A. (1969). *Lancet*, **1**, 307.
3 Riley, I. D. (1969). *Lancet*, **1**, 373.
4 Wheeldon, R. and Heggarty, H. J. (1971). *Arch. Dis. Child*, **46**, 562.
5 Leader (1973). *Brit. med. J.*, **2**, 678.
6 Ginsburg, C. M. (1973). *Am. J. Dis. Child.*, **125**, 241.

CHAPTER 20

MISCELLANEOUS DRUGS

Oral Diuretics

These preparations are widely prescribed for symptomatic relief of fluid retention. Acute poisoning with them is, however, uncommon.

Thiadiazine derivatives form the largest group of diuretic compounds, and there are numerous proprietary preparations available, many of which are mixtures. These drugs are well absorbed from the gastrointestinal tract and their diuretic action begins within an hour of ingestion. The drugs themselves are excreted from three to six hours later. Accompanying the loss of sodium and chloride there is, even in therapeutic doses, a significant potassium loss. Electrolyte imbalance is therefore a prominent feature of overdosage.

Other commonly prescribed non-thiazide diuretics, such as chlorthalidone (Hygroton), triamterene (Dytac), ethacrynic acid (Edecrin) and frusemide (Lasix) have different durations of action from the thiazides but the toxic effects when taken in overdosage are similar.

Clinical Features

Hypersensitivity reactions, which sometimes occur with normal dosage, may also be evident when these drugs are taken in acute overdosage. Skin rashes and photosensitivity may result. Purpura and marrow depression also are found.

The major clinical feature of overdosage is polyuria, the severity of which depends largely on the amount of drug taken. As a result the patient may become dehydrated and develop hypokalaemic hypochloraemic alkalaemia which may be severe. Hypokalaemia may be particularly significant if

146

the patient is being treated with digitalis and if it develops rapidly may result in signs of acute digitalis toxicity (p. 134).

With massive overdosage, or more commonly, if the patient has severe renal disease, acute renal failure with oliguria may occur. Likewise if there is severe pre-existing hepatic disorder acute liver failure may be precipitated although the reason for this is obscure. In susceptible patients an acute attack of gout may be provoked even in a patient who has not been known to have the gouty diathesis.

Biochemical Features

Hyponatraemia.
Hypochloraemia.
Hypokalaemia.
Alkalaemia.
High plasma uric acid.
Mild hyperglycaemia.

Treatment

1. Intensive supportive therapy (p. 18) particularly directed to correction of fluid, electrolyte and acid-base imbalance.
2. Potassium supplements—potassium chloride (2 g) orally three-hourly depending on the degree of hypokalaemia. Digitalis toxicity (p. 135) may require appropriate treatment.
3. Acute attacks of gout should be treated with phenylbutazone 200 mg eight-hourly until the inflammatory changes have subsided.

Antihistamines

This group of drugs is prescribed for a wide variety of conditions including allergies, 'colds', motion sickness and Parkinson's disease. Overdosage is therefore not uncommon. A further significant factor, especially with regard to children, is that these drugs are frequently presented as attractive syrups and elixirs.

Antihistamine drugs are well absorbed following oral administration and also from parenteral sites, or by topical application. After oral administration peak blood levels are reached in about one hour, and rapid hepatic detoxication occurs by hydroxylation and conjugation. Little, if any unchanged drug appears in the urine.

Clinical Features

Antihistamine drugs in acute overdosage produce complex clinical signs which result from both excitation and depression of the central nervous system. In young children the excitatory effects are more prominent. This is further complicated by the fact that the various antihistamines differ in their main toxic effects. For example, diphenhydramine and antazoline have a more marked hypnotic effect than the other members of the group. Moreover some preparations presented under a particular proprietary name are in fact mixtures of different antihistamines. For these reasons, assessment of the severity of the poisonings must depend on the clinical findings. There is considerable individual variation in response to these drugs.

CENTRAL NERVOUS SYSTEM. Drowsiness, headache, blurred vision, tinnitus, urinary retention, and nervousness, are the commonest features of poisoning. In a large overdosage, fixed dilated pupils, disorientation, ataxia, hallucinations, stupor and coma occur. Sometimes an excitatory effect predominates, resulting in hyper-reflexia, tremors, excitement, nystagmus and convulsions.

CARDIOVASCULAR SYSTEM. Hypotension, tachycardia, and occasionally cardiac arrhythmias occur.

RESPIRATORY SYSTEM. Respiratory depression is a feature of severe overdosage.

GASTROINTESTINAL SYSTEM. Dryness of mouth, nausea, and constipation are common.

METABOLIC DISORDER. Hyperpyrexia occurs particularly in children.

EFFECTS ON SKIN. Rashes may be very varied.

BLOOD FINDINGS. Agranulocytosis and aplastic anaemia may develop.

Treatment

1. The principles of intensive supportive therapy (p. 18) should be followed.

2. As the active drug is rapidly metabolised and very little is recovered in the urine, methods to hasten elimination of these preparations are of little value and should not be used.

3. If central nervous stimulation is marked, sedation may be necessary, preferably using diazepam or sodium phenobarbitone by intramuscular injection.

4. If agranulocytosis and aplastic anaemia develop prophylactic antibiotics, adrenocorticosteroid drugs or blood transfusion should be given as circumstances demand.

Oral Anticoagulants

The coumarin and indandione drugs all have similar actions in depressing blood coagulation. They reduce the plasma prothrombin level and depress also factors VII, IX and X[1, 2]. There are many proprietary preparations, the commonest ones used being bishydroxycoumarin (Dicumarol), warfarin (Coumadin, Panwarfarin, Prothromadin), phenindione (Danilone, Dindevan, Hedulin). Acute toxicity may result from excessive therapeutic dosage but in children accidental ingestion of the tablets may occur and in adults they are occasionally taken for purposes of self-poisoning. Warfarin is the main ingredient of many rodenticides and acute overdosage may result from the ingestion of these, accidental or otherwise.

Clinical Features

Bruising and haematemesis and occasionally bleeding elsewhere, such as haematuria and haemoptysis[3]. Orange yellow urine. Diagnosis is confirmed by the finding of a prolonged prothrombin time in the absence of hepatic disorder.

This test is also an index of the severity of the poisoning and of the adequacy of Vitamin K_1 therapy.

Treatment

1. Gastric aspiration and lavage (p. 23).
2. Vitamin K_1 (25 mg) intravenously, repeated as necessary.
3. If haemorrhage is severe, blood transfusion may be required.

Antibiotics

The toxic effects of antibiotics are usually due to either hypersensitivity or are the result of chronic administration. Acute overdosage with antibiotics is relatively uncommon. Poisoning with streptomycin, neomycin, kanamycin, viomycin or vancomycin may damage the eighth nerve with resultant deafness. Toxic effects are likely to be particularly severe if the patient has renal impairment. Cycloserine in acute overdosage produces lethargy, psychotic behaviour, impaired consciousness and coma; convulsions may also occur.

Treatment

1. Intensive supportive therapy (p. 18).
2. Severe sensitivity and anaphylactoid reactions should be treated with corticosteroids.
3. Simple symptomatic treatment is usually all that is necessary. Haemodialysis or peritoneal dialysis has been recommended in severe poisonings with renal impairment, especially in the case of streptomycin, neomycin, kanamycin, gentamycin, viomycin and vancomycin, but these procedures do not prevent toxic damage to the eighth nerve.

Contraceptive 'Pills'

These preparations of sex hormones are fairly frequently taken by inquisitive toddlers. Mild nausea or even vomiting may be produced. Withdrawal bleeding in girls seldom occurs.

Bromides

The bromide salts are steadily losing favour in therapeutics, but their presence in sedative mixtures occasionally results in their being taken in overdosage.

The fatal dose is probably only a few grams, but death very seldom occurs because the drug almost always causes vomiting.

Clinical Features

Nausea and vomiting.
Depression of respiration.
Muscular weakness and paralysis.
Impaired consciousness.
A blood bromide above 60 mg/100 ml.

Treatment

1. Gastric aspiration and lavage (p. 23).
2. Intensive supportive therapy (p. 18).
3. Intravenous infusion of alternating 500 ml N. Saline and 1,000 ml 5 per cent dextrose at a rate of 1,000 ml every two hours until the blood bromide level is below 60 mg per 100 ml[1, 2]. To each 500 ml of the infusion regimen 0·5 g KCl (13 mEq. K^+) should be added. Close biochemical monitoring is essential.
4. Intravenous frusemide (Lasix) 80 mg, repeated in four hours. Regimens adding diuretics such as frusemide or ethacrynic acid and mannitol to the above saline/dextrose infusion regimen have been found to be successful[3], but with these biochemical control is even more important and the patients must be fully hydrated at the beginning of treatment.
5. In patients with cardiac or renal failure haemodialysis is indicated as the above treatments would be hazardous[1].

Thallium

The use of Thallium is steadily increasing in industry but it is as a constituent of rodenticides and insecticides that it is usually a cause of acute poisoning. It may be ingested following contamination of food or from the hands, and it may be inhaled or absorbed through the skin.

Clinical Features

The clinical pattern of acute poisoning follows a rather typical course[1]. Acute vomiting and diarrhoea, which may contain blood, appear within two days and these symptoms usually subside. Within 10 days, however, retrosternal pain and bizarre neurological features resembling the Guillain-Barré syndrome develop. Convulsions, psychosis and tachycardia usually precede the rapid onset of alopecia which occurs from the 15th to 20th day. Death may result from respiratory failure[2, 3].

Thallium is readily detected in the urine throughout the illness and for some time after recovery. Severe poisoning is likely when the urinary secretion of thallium exceeds 10 mg/24 hours.

Treatment

This is difficult. Efforts should be made to increase urinary and faecal excretion.

1. Intensive supportive therapy (p. 18).
2. Potassium chloride 5·0 g orally daily appears to be effective by mobilising thallium from the tissues thereby releasing it for urinary excretion.
3. Activated charcoal may be given orally to inactivate thallium excreted into the intestine.
4. Prussian Blue adsorbs thallium in the gut better than charcoal. Prussian Blue in 'solution' 250 mg per kg per day should be given orally, if necessary through a duodenal tube. The appropriate dose should be given six-hourly. To each dose there should be added 50 ml of 15 per cent mannitol. This therapy should be continued until the urinary excretion of thallium does not exceed 0·5 mg in 24 hours[4, 5].
5. Various chelating agents such as dithiocarb and dithizone have been advocated, but their disadvantage is that the

chelate reaches the brain more readily than thallium ion, thereby worsening the condition[3].

Prognosis

Complete recovery can occur, but there are often residual defects such as ataxia, foot drop and optic atrophy.

Oral Hypoglycaemic Agents

These preparations are used widely in the treatment of diabetes mellitus and they are readily available in the community. It is not surprising, therefore, that they are quite commonly involved in acute poisoning incidents. In children the overdosage is usually accidental but in adults the great majority are self-poisonings. Acute toxicity may result from the ingestion of comparatively few tablets.

The Biguanides

These include phenformin (Dibotin) and metformin (Glucophage, Diguanil, Metiguanide).

Clinical Features

ALIMENTARY SYSTEM.   Nausea and vomiting are common and so much of the ingested dose may be eliminated. Abdominal pain may be followed by haematemesis and melaena.

CENTRAL NERVOUS SYSTEM.   Depressed limb reflexes but with bilateral extensor plantar responses. Drowsiness proceeding rapidly to coma, which may be severe. Muscular twitching and convulsions.

RESPIRATORY SYSTEM.   Hyperpnoea which is usually Kussmaul in type. Acute pulmonary oedema is a common cause of death in this poisoning.

CARDIOVASCULAR SYSTEM.   Tachycardia. Hypotension and 'shock' which may be severe.

METABOLIC DISORDER.   Absence of sweating is characteristic. Hypoglycaemia with a blood sugar often less than 25 mg

154 TREATMENT OF COMMON ACUTE POISONINGS

per 100 ml. Hyperkalaemia. Acidosis due to lactic acidaemia is often marked[1, 2].

A high neutrophil leucocytosis may be present.

Treatment

1. Intensive supportive therapy (p. 18).
2. Glucagon 1 mg intravenously, supplemented if necessary by intravenous glucose (50 ml of 50 per cent solution of dextrose) to correct hypoglycaemia.
3. Sodium bicarbonate in appropriate doses to correct acidaemia. This may prove difficult but the administration of intravenous methylene blue is a helpful addition[3].
4. Correction of electrolyte upset.

The Sulphonylureas

This group of drugs includes tolbutamide (Rastinon, Artosin, Orimase, D.860) and chlorpropamide (Diabinase). The effective action of tolbutamide does not exceed 6 to 8 hours, whereas the biological half-life of chlorpropamide is 36 hours[4]. The latter drug is the most commonly prescribed sulphonylurea and also the one most frequently a cause of overdosage.

The clinical features of poisoning are similar to those of the biguanides but gastrointestinal upsets are less. In view of the prolonged action of chlorpropamide, correction of the profound hypoglycaemia requires not only large doses of glucagon and intravenous glucose, but also repeated administration[4, 5, 6].

REFERENCES

Anticoagulants

1 Lowenthal, J. and MacFarlane, J. A. (1967). *J. Pharmac. exp. Ther.*, **157**, 672.
2 Lowenthal, J. and Birnbaum, H. (1968). *Science, N.Y.*, **164**, 181.
3 Levine, W. G. (1970). Anticoagulants. In *The Pharmacological Basis of Therapeutics*, ed. Goodman, L. S. and Gilman, A., p. 1451. New York: Collier.

Bromides

1 Wieth, J. O. and Funder, J. (1963). *Lancet*, **2**, 327.
2 Nuki, G., Richardson, P., Goggin, M. J. and Bayliss, R. I. S. (1966). *Brit. med. J.*, **2**, 390.
3 Adamson, J. S., Flanigan, W. J. and Ackerman, G. L. (1966). *Ann. Intern. Med.*, **65**, 749.

Thallium

1 Bank, W. J., Pleasure, D. E., Suzuki, K., Nigro, M. and Katz, R. (1972). *Arch. Neurol.*, **26**, 456.
2 Leader, *Brit. med. J.* (1972). **3**, 717.
3 Cavanagh, J. B., Fuller, N. H., Johnson, H. R. M. and Rudge, P. (1974). *Quart. J. med.*, N.S., **43**, 293.
4 Kamerbeek, H. H. (1972). *Clin. Toxicol.*, **5**, 90.
5 Kamerbeek, H. H., Rouws, A. G., ten Ham, M. and van Heijst, A. N. (1971). *Acta Medica Scand.*, **89**, 321.

Oral Hypoglycaemics

1 Sadow, H. S. (1969). *Postgrad. med. J.*, **45**, *Suppl.*, p. 30.
2 Bingle, T. P., Storey, G. W. and Winter, J. M. (1970). *Brit. med. J.*, **3**, 752.
3 Tranquada, R. E., Grant, W. J. and Peterson, C. R. (1966). *Arch. Int. med.*, **117**, 192.
4 Dowell, R. C. and Imrie, A. A. (1972). *Scot. med. J.*, **17**, 305.
5 Davies, D. M., MacIntyre, A. Millar, J., Bell, S. M. and Mehra, S. K. (1967). *Lancet*, **1**, 363.
6 Forrest, J. A. H. (1974). *Clin. Toxicol.*, **7**, 19.

L

CHAPTER 21

MISCELLANEOUS DOMESTIC AND INDUSTRIAL SUBSTANCES

Most poisonings due to these substances are truly accidental and in the case of household preparations are most common in children.

Bleaches

BLEACH CONTAINING SODIUM HYPOCHLORITE

Household bleaching solutions—so frequently left under the kitchen sink and therefore available to the toddler—contain about 5 per cent sodium hypochlorite. They are corrosive in themselves and this becomes more so because hypochlorous acid is released on contact with gastric HCl. During this reaction evolution of free chlorine gas occurs in the stomach. This may then be inhaled with resultant pulmonary damage. Hypochlorous acid is, however, of low toxicity after absorption.

Clinical Features

If inhaled: Cough and possible pulmonary oedema.

If ingested: Irritation of mouth and pharynx.

                  Oedema of the pharynx and larynx.

                  Nausea and vomiting.

If in contact with skin: local irritation.

Treatment

1. Gastric aspiration, and lavage with appropriate volumes of 2·5 per cent sodium thiosulphate. If sodium thiosulphate is not available use copious amounts of milk of magnesia in water or milk itself.

2. If severely ill sodium thiosulphate (1 per cent) 250 ml intravenously.

BLEACH CONTAINING OXALIC ACID

This form of bleach is used also as a metal cleaner. The fatal dose is in the region of 5 g. The toxic effects give rise to muscular hyperexcitability and convulsions. These result from hypocalcaemia due to the essentially irreversible combination of oxalate with plasma calcium. Death may occur in a few minutes.

Clinical Features

GASTROINTESTINAL SYSTEM. Irritation of mouth and throat. Nausea and vomiting.

CENTRAL NERVOUS SYSTEM. Muscular twitchings and convulsions.

CARDIOVASCULAR SYSTEM. Shock and cardiac arrest.

RENAL DISORDER. Acute renal failure, the development of which may occur some time after apparent clinical recovery.

Treatment

1. Gastric aspiration and lavage (p. 23) adding 10 g calcium lactate to lavage fluid and leaving 100 ml 1 per cent calcium lactate in stomach.
2. Intensive supportive therapy (p. 18).
3. Calcium gluconate 10 per cent, 10 ml intravenously and repeat if features of severe poisoning persist.
4. Provided the renal output is adequate at least 5 litres of fluid should be given for three days. This will help to prevent precipitation of calcium oxalate in the renal tubules.

Chlorate

Sodium or potassium chlorate salts are contained in many gargles and lozenges. Sodium chlorate is used as a weed killer. The potentially fatal dose in an adult is approximately 15 g. The chief effects are irritation of the alimentary system. Severe methaemoglobinaemia may occur. Renal and liver damage are likely after ingestion of a large quantity.

Clinical Features

GASTROINTESTINAL SYSTEM. Nausea, vomiting, colic and diarrhoea. Jaundice and hepatic failure.

BLOOD FINDINGS. Haemolysis. Methaemoglobinaemia which may reach 40 per cent or more, which is a dangerous level.

RENAL DISORDERS. Blood, protein and haemoglobin products may be present in the urine. Oliguria or anuria.

CENTRAL NERVOUS SYSTEM. The initial confusion may be followed by coma and convulsions.

LABORATORY FINDINGS. Methaemoglobinaemia. Haemolysis. Raised serum potassium.

Treatment

1. Intensive supportive therapy (p. 18).
2. If cyanosis is severe, methylene blue 25 ml of 1 per cent solution slowly intravenously. If methylene blue is not available ascorbic acid, 1 g slowly intravenously.
3. Forced diuresis if urinary output is adequate (p. 35).
4. Haemodialysis or peritoneal dialysis (p. 36) is valuable in severe poisoning.
5. Hepatic and renal failure may require conventional treatment.

Phenol, Lysol and Cresol

These compounds are in common use as potent antiseptics particularly as washing fluids. Acute poisoning, although at one time quite common, is now seldom found. The toxic effects are however severe but with appropriate treatment can often be prevented or alleviated.

Phenol compounds are readily absorbed by all routes and can even enter the body in toxic quantities through contact with the intact skin. About 80 per cent of the chemical is excreted through the kidney either as the active principle or else as the glucuronide or sulphate.

Clinical Features

In this poisoning there is usually a strong smell of carbolic acid in the patient's breath or vomit.

GASTROINTESTINAL SYSTEM. When taken orally, corrosive changes on the lips and buccal mucosa result. The patient complains of surprisingly little pain in these ulcers, as the poison is so corrosive that it destroys the nerve endings in the burnt areas. There can be, however, abdominal pain, nausea, and vomiting, and life-threatening gastric haemorrhage or perforation may occur. If the patient recovers, strictures, especially in the oesophagus are likely.

CENTRAL NERVOUS SYSTEM. After absorption, there may be an initial phase of excitement which progresses to impaired level of consciousness.

CARDIOVASCULAR SYSTEM. Hypotension and 'shock' are common.

RENAL DISORDERS. The urine is dark due to free haemoglobin. Oliguria, anuria and renal failure may develop.

HEPATIC DISORDER. Damage may be severe and result in acute liver failure.

RESPIRATORY SYSTEM. In severe cases respiratory depression is prominent and respiratory failure is a common cause of death.

HAEMOPOIETIC SYSTEM. Cyanosis may occur due to methaemoglobinaemia.

Treatment

1. Gastric aspiration and lavage (p. 23) should be done in all cases with caution, as every effort must be made to reduce absorption to the minimum. Castor oil or olive oil will dissolve phenol and delay absorption and, so, if these are available, one or other should be added to the lavage fluid.
2. Intensive supportive therapy (p. 18).

3. If phenol has come into contact with the skin this should be washed either with copious water or 50 per cent alcohol.
4. Routine medical measures for renal failure and, if these fail, haemodialysis may be considered.
5. When methaemoglobinaemia is marked, methylene blue should be given slowly intravenously (25ml of 1 per cent solution) and repeated as necessary.

Naphthalene

Naphthalene may be taken by children when air freshener discs or old fashioned mothballs are eaten. About 2 g is a fatal dose for a small child, as absorption occurs rapidly. Haemolysis with subsequent renal failure is the chief danger. Liver necrosis may also occur. Paradichlorbenzene which is the main ingredient of many modern moth repellants is considerably less toxic.

Clinical Features

GASTROINTESTINAL SYSTEM. Nausea, vomiting and diarrhoea. Jaundice and liver failure may follow.

HAEMATOLOGICAL SYSTEM. Anaemia due to haemolysis.

RENAL DISORDERS. Oliguria, haematuria and proteinuria.

CENTRAL NERVOUS SYSTEM. Cerebral stimulation, with agitation leading to coma and convulsions.

Treatment

1. Gastric aspiration and lavage (p. 23).
2. Alkalinise the urine with oral sodium bicarbonate, or if this is not retained, intravenous sodium bicarbonate, 500 ml (1·25 per cent).
3. Hydrocortisone (100 mg) six-hourly intramuscularly.
4. Blood transfusions if haemolysis is severe.
5. Oliguria or anuria may require intensive medical treatment and haemodialysis, if this is ineffective.

Detergents

Apart from producing nausea, vomiting and diarrhoea, the common household detergents are not toxic.

Metaldehyde

This is a constituent of snail bait and certain firelighters. Occasionally it is sampled by children. It is a polymer of acetaldehyde and its toxic effects appear to be due to this substance. Common features of poisoning include nausea and intractable vomiting, hyper-reflexia, convulsions, respiratory depression and circulatory collapse.

Treatment

This consists of gastric aspiration and lavage and intensive supportive therapy (p. 18).

Matches

Children may on occasion chew or swallow matches. Little upset is likely other than nausea, vomiting and diarrhoea if less than six have been taken by a 3 year old toddler. There are two main types of matchheads in common use. Friction matchheads contain phosphorus whereas the heads of safety matches have the following constituents, potassium chlorate, antimony trioxide and sulphur, and the phosphorus is on the striking surface of the box. If a child ingests safety matches it is most unlikely that there will be any ill-effect apart from mild alimentary upset. When friction matches are taken mild phosphorus poisoning may result (p. 126).

Turpentine

Turpentine is often considered to be a cause of poisoning in children, but in the United Kingdom, at least, it is unusual for pure turpentine to be available: turpentine substitute (white spirit) is almost always the household preparation. It is important to distinguish these as the toxic effects are different. Turpentine substitute has been described (p. 62).

Clinical Features

GASTROINTESTINAL SYSTEM. Nausea, vomiting, colic, diarrhoea.

CENTRAL NERVOUS SYSTEM. Excitement, delirium, convulsions, coma.

RESPIRATORY SYSTEM. Central depression. Pneumonia.

RENAL DISORDERS. Albuminuria, haematuria and renal failure may occur.

Treatment

1. Intensive supportive therapy (p. 18) including gastric aspiration and lavage in contrast to turpentine substitute.
2. Renal failure may require conventional treatment.

CHAPTER 22

VENOMOUS ANIMALS

Acute poisoning due to this cause is commonest in tropical and subtropical climates. The precise chemical composition and pathophysiology of animal venoms is incompletely known and so the range of specific treatment is limited[1]. The general principles of intensive supportive therapy (p. 18) should be followed in the management of these poisonings as is the case with drug overdosage.

Snakebite

There are over 2,000 species of snake in the world, but only about 250 are venomous. Poisonous snakes may be divided into four main groups according to the type of fang which they possess[1].

Family	Common Names
Crotalidae	Rattlesnakes
	Pit vipers
Viperidae	True viper
Elapidae	Cobras
	Kraits
	Mambas
Hydrophidae	Sea snakes

Every year 30,000 people die from snakebites in the world, the great majority being in India and South-East Asia. In Europe the mortality is less than 1 per cent of the total and in the United Kingdom deaths from this cause are rare. Snake bites occur most often in children, who have disturbed the snakes as a result of curiosity, or in men, who have disturbed them in the course of their work.

Snake venoms contain enzymes, non-enzymatic proteins and other substances such as acetyl choline and 5-hydroxy-tryptamine[2]. Apart from the direct effects of these compounds they also provoke tissue production of other inflammatory agents such as kinins, histamines and slow reacting substance[3, 4]. The severity of the toxic effects of snake bite depend on the type and quantity of venom injected. This in turn depends on the age, size and sex of the snake and bites occurring at night are more venomous than during the day. In the case of hibernating snakes, the venom is particularly potent just after hibernation is over.

Clinical Features

Venomous snakes leave characteristically two or occasionally one fang mark, whereas bites from non-poisonous snakes produce a semi-circular set of tooth marks.

(a) *Local Effects*. These may be of no more than a mild inflammatory reaction or slight bruising. Tissue necrosis is particularly likely, however, in bites from *Viperidae* and *Crotalidae*[5]. The necrosis occurs several days after the bite, but is preceded by marked pain and swelling.

(b) *Systemic Effects*. Venom from *Crotalidae*, *Viperidae* and *Elapidae* may cause the following effects.

GASTROINTESTINAL SYSTEM. Nausea and vomiting.

CARDIOVASCULAR SYSTEM. Hypotension is common due to vasodilatation and hypovolaemia[6].

CENTRAL NERVOUS SYSTEM. Drowsiness, muscular weakness, which may result in diplopia and difficulty with speech and swallowing. In severe cases ventilatory paralysis may occur, and coma and convulsions may develop. Sensory function remains normal[3].

HAEMATOLOGICAL SYSTEM. Increased blood coagulability may result from rattlesnake bite, whereas with the Malayan Pit Viper a prolonged coagulation defect with extensive ecchymoses and general bleeding tendency may occur due to a very low plasma fibrinogen[7, 8].

Sea snake bites characteristically result in marked poly-myositis with a 'limb-girdle' distribution. Muscle enzymes and plasma potassium levels are elevated and myoglobinuria with renal failure may occur. The muscle damage is so severe that patients may have marked weakness for several months[9].

Treatment

There are a number of popular misconceptions regarding the management of snake bite[10]. There is no evidence that there is any value in the use of tourniquets[5] or incision and suction of the injection site[11], and in unskilled hands these maneouvres may be even harmful. Cooling of the bite area, the administration of antihistamines[12] and corticosteroids[13] have all been advocated but none of these are considered helpful now in snake bite. These methods of treatment, therefore, should be avoided. Recommended treatment consists of:

1. Careful cleansing of the wound with sterile saline or water.
2. Immobilisation is valuable treatment, particularly for the local effects.
3. Intensive supportive therapy (p. 18).
4. Inject tetanus antitoxin or, if the victim has previously been inoculated against tetanus, a booster dose of tetanus toxoid.
5. Inject crystalline penicillin 2 mega units intramuscularly.
6. Sedation and analgesics may be required as the instictive reaction to snake bite is fear of rapid death.
7. ANTIVENINS. As snake venoms are largely protein, they are antigenic and antivenins can be prepared from horse serum. Many antivenins are polyvalent containing anti-bodies to several venoms. They are ineffective to certain viper and elapidine venoms, and often provoke serious allergic reactions which may be fatal[1]. Their use, therefore, must be considered very carefully. In the United Kingdom, for example, the only poisonous snake is the adder (*Vipera berus*) and authoritative opinion (Royal Society of Tropical Medicine and Hygiene) states that the effects of the vipera

berus bite is less dangerous than the use of the antivenin and this should *not* be used, except in the very unusual severely ill patient when Zagreb antivenin should be given by intravenous drip.

Antivenins are indicated only when systemic effects develop or when extensive local tissue damage is present[3]. A test dose should always be given before administering the full therapeutic dose. Reid has shown that antivenin is helpful in cobra bite[5] and in the case of the Malayan Pit Viper a specific antivenin has produced a very significant reduction in mortality[13]. In sea snake bite there is also a specific antivenin and its use will avoid the prolonged muscle weakness, which occurs in that poisoning[15]. Haemodialysis has also been advocated in sea snake bite and it is claimed that apart from treating renal failure the muscle weakness is improved[16].

Insect Bites

Stings from ants, bees, wasps and hornets seldom cause severe toxic effects apart from local pain and swelling, unless the bite is on the mouth or tongue when the associated swelling may cause respiratory distress. Rarely deaths have been reported from very extensive stings or more commonly due to severe allergic reactions, especially to bee stings. Bee stings are alkaline and wasp, hornet and ant stings are acid and the appropriate application of an acid or alkaline solution respectively is usually all that is necessary. If the local reaction is marked an antihistamine given systemically is helpful. In severe allergic reactions subcutaneous adrenaline 1:1000 (0·5 ml) and hydrocortisone 100 mg intravenously may be life-saving.

Spider Bites

Spiders poisonous to man live in warm climates. The Black Widow Spider (*Lactrodectus mactans*) and the Funnel Web Spider (*Atrax robustus*) are quite frequent causes of poisonous bites. They commonly inhabit outhouses, basements and foundations of houses and outside lavatories. Children and workmen are most often the victims. Death occurs in up to 6 per cent of cases, especially in young children.

Clinical Features

The initial bite may be unnoticed. Within about an hour, however, the following occur.

LOCOMOTOR DISORDERS. Generalised muscular pains and stiffness. Burning sensation of feet.

GASTROINTESTINAL SYSTEM. Nausea and vomiting. If there is marked abdominal rigidity a mistaken diagnosis of peritonitis may be made. Salivation.

METABOLIC DISORDERS. Pyrexia and sweating.

Leucocytosis, mild hypertension and a macular rash may also occur.

Treatment

1. Cleanse the bite with sterile saline or water.
2. Analgesics for relief of pain. 10-20 ml of 10 per cent calcium gluconate by slow intravenous injection.
3. If secondary infection occurs systemic antibiotics.
4. Intensive supportive therapy (p. 18).
5. If the systemic features are severe administer the specific antivenin, if this is available.

In the more Southern States of America and Mexico the Brown Recluse Spider (*Loxosceles reclusa*) and associated species are common. The incidence of poisoning by this venomous spider is relatively low, but the condition is generally regarded as serious as the necrotic ulcer which results is very slow to heal and is prone to form extensive scar tissue. The bite may be symptomless for several hours and then is followed by acute pain and subsequent tissue necrosis. Medical treatment has failed to influence the course of the condition apart from prevention of secondary infection. Surgical excision of the affected area within four to six hours may help to limit the tissue necrosis.

Scorpions

These nocturnal creatures live in the tropics or sub-tropics. The sting is rarely fatal.

Clinical Features

Marked local pain occurs after the sting[18]. Subsequently sweating, numbness and hyperaesthesiae may develop. In severe cases, central respiratory and cardiac depression may be marked.

Treatment

1. Cleanse the sting.
2. Analgesics for the pain.
3. Intensive supportive therapy (p. 18).

Venomous Sea Animals

Poisoning by sea snakes has been described (p. 165).

STING RAYS (*Urobatis Halleri*)

These fish live in warm seas and they present a hazard usually to bathers, who inadvertantly stand on the fish lying in the sand. The venom contains a thermolabile toxin. Fatalities are uncommon and usually result from extensive injury, especially if the sting sheath remains in the wound[19].

Clinical Features

Usually the sting results in a jagged wound and severe local pain[20]. Systemic features may develop and include hypotension, oculogyric crises and convulsions.

Treatment

Incision and suction of the wound should *not* be done.
1. Careful cleansing of the wound with surgical exploration if the sting sheath has been retained. The wound should be immersed in the hottest water bearable in an attempt to destroy the toxin. Local anaesthetic, systemic analgesics and corticosteroids are often helpful[21].
2. Intensive supportive therapy (p. 18) in severe cases.

In British waters there are two species of Weaver Fish (*Trachinus*) which are found off the shores of Cornwall. These have sharp dorsal and opercular spines which may cause wounds and toxic effects similar to sting rays.

JELLYFISH

In the seas around the United Kingdom the majority of jellyfish are harmless to humans. Those which can sting include the blue *Cyanea lamareki* and the yellow *Cyanea capillata*[22], which have a lobulated bell and eight tufts of long tentacles, and the large *Chrysaora isosceles* with radiating bands of white and brown from the centre of its bell and 24 long tentacles. Occasionally the Portuguese Man-of-War (*physalia*), which has a blue float and very long tentacles, enters British waters.

Clinical Features

Local pain is the main effect. Physalia stings are more severe[22] and pain may be very marked and generalised muscle pains, colic, nausea and breathlessness with cyanosis may result. Death from Physalia stings may occur rapidly within minutes or be delayed for some hours.

Treatment

1. Any tentacles still adherent to the bather must be removed with care, preferably by adhesive tape, and on no account should they be brushed off with a bare hand as the tentacles may be still capable of delivering a sting for many hours after removal from the water.
2. Analgesics for pain. Local anaesthetic creams are effective.
3. Intensive supportive therapy (p. 18) if systemic features are prominent.

Another jellyfish with a potentially lethal sting is the sea wasp (*Chiropsalmus quadrigatus*) which lives in the seas off North-East Australia.

REFERENCES

Venomous Animals

1 George, C. F. (1972). *Medicine*, **4**, 317.
2 Jimenez-Porras, J. M. (1970). *Clinical Toxicology*, **3**, 389.
3 Meldrum, B. S. (1965). *Pharmac. Revs.*, **17**, 393.
4 Russell, F. E. and Puffer, H. W. (1970). *Clin. Toxicology*, **3**, 433.
5 Reid, H. A. (1964). *Brit. med. J.*, **2**, 540.
6 Halmagyi, D. F. J., Starzecki, B. and Horner, G. J. (1965). *J. Appl. Physiol.*, **20**, 709.
7 Reid, H. A., Chan, K. E. and Thean, P. C. (1963). *Lancet*, **1**, 621.
8 Reid, H. A., Thean, P. C., Chan, K. E. and Baharom, A. R. (1963). *Lancet*, **1**, 617.
9 Reid, H. A. (1961). *Lancet*, **2**, 399.
10 Reid, H. A. (1970). *Clin. Toxicology*, **3**, 473.
11 Ya, P. M. and Perry, J. F. (1960). *Surgery (St. Louis)*, **47**, 975.
12 Stimson, A. C. and Engelhardt, H. T. (1960). *J. Occup. Med.*, **2**, 163.
13 Reid, H. A., Thean, P. C. and Martin, W. J. (1963). *Brit. med. J.*, **2**, 1378.
14 Leading article (1969). *Brit. med. J.*, **3**, 370.
15 Reid, H. A. (1962). *Brit. med. J.*, **2**, 576.
16 Sitprija, V., Sribhibhadh, R. and Benyahati, C. (1971). *Brit. med. J.*, **3**, 218.
17 Butz, W. C. (1971). *Clin. Toxicology*, **4**, 515.
18 Yarom, R. (1970). *Clin. Toxicology*, **3**, 561.
19 Russell, F. E., Panos, T. C., Kang, L. W., Warner, A. M. and Colket, T. C. (1958). *Amer. J. med. Sci.*, **235**, 566.
20 Russell, F. E. (1953). *Amer. J. med. Sci.*, **226**, 611.
21 Mullaney, P. J. (1970). *Clin. Toxicology*, **3**, 613.
22 Southcott, R. V. (1970). *Clin. Toxicology*, **3**, 617.

CHAPTER 23

INSECTICIDES AND HERBICIDES

The common insecticides and herbicides fall into the following groups:

1. Phenolic substances, e.g., dinitro-ortho-cresol; dinitrophenol.
2. Organophosphorous compounds, e.g., parathion; tepp; malathion.
3. Paraquat, e.g., gramoxone; gramixel; priglone; wecdol.
4. Arsenicals (p. 119).

Due to stringent and carefully enforced legislation regarding their use poisoning with these substances is fortunately not frequently seen in the United Kingdom, in spite of their toxicity.

Dinitro-Ortho-Cresol and Dinitrophenol

Various formulations of these substances are used in agriculture. They are usually supplied as concentrates which require to be diluted before use. It is during this process that they are likely to come into contact with the skin: a characteristic yellow staining results. Inhalation and ingestion may occur during spraying of crops. In the human body poisoning results primarily from their uncoupling action which leads to a great increase in cellular metabolism. They are especially dangerous in hot climates when the body already has difficulty in losing heat.

The features of acute poisoning develop either after a single large dose, or else after chronic exposure when a critical threshold has been reached.

171

Clinical Features

These may develop with alarming suddenness and resemble a thyrotoxic crisis.

CENTRAL NERVOUS SYSTEM. Anxiety, restlessness, tiredness, insomnia, convulsions and coma.

CARDIOVASCULAR SYSTEM. Tachycardia and arrhythmias.

RESPIRATORY SYSTEM. Tachypnoea and pulmonary congestion.

METABOLIC DISORDERS. Hyperpyrexia and intense perspiration.

EFFECTS ON SKIN. Burns of lips and buccal mucosa. Yellow staining of exposed skin.

RENAL DISORDER. Acute renal failure may develop.

HEPATIC DISORDER. Acute liver necrosis occurs.

A blood dinitro-ortho-cresol level above 5 mg per 100 ml indicates severe poisoning.

Treatment

1. Remove from exposure and then keep at complete rest. Wash the yellow skin, which does not remove the yellow staining but prevents further absorption.
2. Intensive supportive therapy (p. 18).
3. Ice packs and fans to reduce body temperature.
4. Sedation with chlorpromazine (100 mg intramuscularly) repeated as necessary.
5. Maintenance of fluids and electrolyte balance by intravenous infusion of appropriate quantities of 5 per cent dextrose and N, saline in rotation.
6. Correct arrhythmias by appropriate drugs under ECG control.

Prognosis

Death may occur in the early stages if treatment is not sufficiently energetic.

Organophosphorous Compounds

These insecticides are very toxic[1] and it is likely that the incidence of poisoning by them will increase as organophosphorous compounds are being used as substitutes for D.D.T. following the ban of that substance in some countries. One drop of undiluted parathion in the eye may be fatal. Poisoning usually occurs from cutaneous absorption, or rarely, by ingestion or inhalation. Their toxicity is due to the inhibition of cholinesterase; the consequent damage can be severe and may not be reversible unless the patient is treated within a few hours.

Clinical Features

Symptoms are usually apparent within two hours of exposure. The diversity of clinical features is likely to lead the physician to think of other conditions especially respiratory or alimentary disease[2]. This is especially so in children when information about the poisoning may be scanty. In adults there is seldom difficulty as most cases result from accidental occupational exposure. Delay in diagnosis can be life-threatening.

RESPIRATORY SYSTEM. Bronchospasm and bronchorrhoea, cyanosis, acute pulmonary oedema; respiratory arrest is the usual cause of death.

CENTRAL NERVOUS SYSTEM. Sweating, lacrimation, headache, restlessness, ataxia, muscle weakness, fibrillary twitching, emotional lability, confusion and convulsions. The pupils may be constricted or widely dilated.

ALIMENTARY SYSTEM. Salivation is an important symptom. Nausea, vomiting, colic and diarrhoea may occur.

CARDIOVASCULAR SYSTEM. Retrosternal tightness, bradycardia, hypotension, peripheral circulatory failure.

LABORATORY FINDINGS. Plasma cholinesterase will be less than 30 per cent of normal.

Treatment

1. Prevent further exposure. Wearing rubber gloves wash skin thoroughly with soap and water, the final swabbing being with ethyl alcohol.

2. Gastric aspiration and lavage if poison has been ingested (p. 23).

3. Intensive supportive therapy (p. 18) with particular emphasis on the maintenance of respiration and correction of cyanosis.

4. As soon as cyanosis is overcome but not before, atropine sulphate (2 mg) should be given intravenously and repeated at 5-10 minute intervals until atropinisation is achieved. Thereafter it is essential to continue an effective level of dosage for at least two or three days. Atropine must *not* be given to a cyanosed patient, lest ventricular fibrillation is inducted. It is not unusual for 50 mg of atropine to be required in the first 24 hours and even 1·5 g have been given to a child in the course of a day. This necessitates considerable quantities of atropine being readily available.

5. Pralidoxime is a specific reactivator of cholinesterase and should be used in addition to atropine[3, 4]. Inject 30 mg/kg (i.e. about 1-2 g) intravenously at a rate not exceeding 500 mg per minute and repeat half-hourly, if necessary. After injecting pralidoxime, the effects of atropine may become more evident and a reduction in the dosage schedule of the latter may be necessary.

6. If sedation or control of convulsions is required, short acting barbiturates may be used but with the greatest caution. Aminophylline, morphine and phenothiazines are contraindicated.

   Note: Supplies of pralidoxime are held at strategic centres. Telephone numbers and addresses may be obtained from the Poisons Information Service.

Paraquat

This herbicide, chemically a dipyridilium, is very toxic in the concentrated liquid form as supplied to farmers and horticulturists[1]. It has the unique property of being inactivated by contact with soil. The brown liquid concentrate usually contains 20 per cent of the active substance in a vehicle which has itself corrosive properties. The granular preparation is available for domestic use and contains 5 per cent of paraquat or di-quat. The granules are dissolved in water prior to application to the weeds. Despite the grim image of paraquat often depicted in the popular press recovery has occurred after ingestion of the concentrated material and there is only one recorded death following ingestion of the granular form. It is, nevertheless, a very serious poisoning with high mortality.

In adults, suicidal poisoning with paraquat concentrate is as common as accidental ingestion. The latter usually occurs from the concentrate being decanted into aerated water bottles, the labels of which are not altered. Children may eat the granules in accidental poisoning or may consume the dregs of a drum which has contained the concentrate.

Clinical Features

ALIMENTARY SYSTEM. A burning sensation in the mouth and abdomen is noticed at the time of ingestion and after a few hours painful ulceration of the lips, tongue and fauces appears. Spontaneous vomiting is unfortunately not common.

RESPIRATORY SYSTEM. Some days, often a week, after ingestion the relentless proliferative alveolitis and terminal bronchiolitis are likely to become evident clinically. These changes may be confirmed by a granular appearance of the lung fields on X-ray[3] and by demonstrating deterioration in respiratory function tests especially in the TCO transference test[4]. It is important, however, to ensure that any deterioration is not due to pulmonary oedema or infection before ascribing it to paraquat lung changes.

RENAL FAILURE. Acute renal failure which is however reversible may occur.

HEPATIC DISORDER. Jaundice with a biochemical pattern of parenchymatous change may be severe but full recovery of function can take place.

CARDIOVASCULAR SYSTEM. Ingestion of a large amount of concentrate will produce severe shock within a very few hours. The shock is probably due to widespread cellular damage and is resistant to treatment. Following ingestion of smaller amounts, pericarditis may develop about the tenth day.

LABORATORY FINDINGS. A simple and sensitive screening test is available[5] and should always be employed to confirm the ingestion of paraquat. A knife tip, about 100 mg sodium hydrogen carbonate, followed by a similar amount of sodium dithionite (hydrosulphite) is added to 5 ml of approximately neutral urine or gastric content. A blue colour develops almost immediately.

Treatment

1. Careful gastric aspiration and lavage (p. 23). Leave 500 ml of 7 per cent bentonite or Fuller's earth suspension in the stomach if paraquat ingested within two hours.
2. Immediate forced diuresis (p. 35) is usually safe at outset before renal damage takes place.
3. Intensive supportive therapy (p. 18).
4. Haemodialysis has not been shown to remove paraquat[2]. This is an exceptional finding for a substance which appears in considerable quantities in the urine. The explanation may be that paraquat is actively secreted by the renal tubules or that paraquat is adsorbed by the dialysis membane.
5. It is likely that paraquat would be removed from the blood by passage through a charcoal column. It is improbable, however, that the removal would have any effect on the proliferative lung lesion which starts within a few hours of ingestion.
6. Attempts at preventing lung changes. As it is thought that the lung lesion is similar to that arising from oxygen

toxicity, attempts have been made to prevent the accumulation of paraquat in the lung. The enzyme superoxidase, d-propranolol and beclomethasone together have all been tried[6]. As yet there is no evidence that paraquat lung changes have been prevented, arrested or reversed by these substances.

Corticosteroids and immunosuppressive drugs do not have any effect in preventing the lung lesion[2].

REFERENCES

Organophosphorous Compounds

1 Namba, T., Nolte, C. T., Jackrel, J. and Grob, D. (1971). *Am. J. Med.*, **50**, 475.
2 Nelson, D. L. and Crawford, C. R. (1972). *Clin. Toxicol.*, **5** (2), 223.
3 Windsor, P. W. M. (1968). *Practitioner*, **200**, 600.
4 Sidell, F. R. (1974). *Clin. Toxicol.*, **7**, 1.

Paraquat

1 Campbell, S. (1968). *Lancet*, **1**, 144.
2 Matthew, H. (1971). *Scot. med. J.*, **16**, 407.
3 Davidson, J. K. and Macpherson, P. (1972). *Clin. Radiol.*, **23**, 18.
4 Cooke, N. J., Flenley, D. C. and Matthew, H. (1973). *Quart. J. Med.*, **42** (168), 683.
5 Tompsett, S. L. (1970). *Acta pharmacol. et toxicol.*, **28**, 346.
6 *Nature* (1973), **245**, 64.

CHAPTER 24

POISONOUS FUNGI, PLANTS, SHRUBS, AND TREES

It is not possible in this chapter to mention poisonous fungi, plants, shrubs and trees to be found throughout the world. The reader should seek information from the poisons information service in his own country or refer to textbooks on the subject [1, 2] (see also Table VIII).

Mushroom Poisoning

Poisonous species of fungi in Britain are very few in number, but danger arises from the fact that they grow wherever edible varieties are to be found. There are no reliable tests to determine whether a mushroom is safe to eat except by expert identification.

AMANITA PHALLOIDES—DEATH CAP

This is a common species found in wooded countryside and it is the most dangerous fungus and accounts for 90 per cent of deaths from this type of poisoning. *A. phalloides* has some resemblance to edible varieties of mushroom, but its cap is usually olive green and silky in appearance, with radiating black fibrils. The gills are white or cream, and there is a cup-like socket at the bottom of the stem. The ingestion of even a small amount of this mushroom may be fatal. The toxin is resistant to heat and may survive cooking.

Clinical Features

The clinical course of poisoning can usually be divided into three phases. There is invariably a latent period between ingestion and the onset of symptoms. This period is seldom shorter than six hours and may be as long as 12 hours.

PHASE 1.—Nausea, vomiting, severe abdominal pains and diarrhoea occur. The diarrhoea may be explosive resembling that of cholera. If the poisoning is severe there will be associated features of collapse.

PHASE 2.—Apparent improvement occurs. This may engender a sense of false security, and recovery may be thought to have taken place.

PHASE 3.—Toxic changes occur in the liver, kidneys, heart and central nervous system. If sufficiently severe, extensive hepatic necrosis occurs characterised by profound abnormalities in liver function tests. Hypoglycaemia also develops. The effect of the toxin on the renal cells is less intensive but there may be proteinuria and impaired creatinine clearance.

On occasions in severe poisoning the three phases may blend into a continuous picture of massive cellular destruction leading rapidly to death.

Treatment

1. There is no specific therapy. An antiphalloidian serum has been produced by immunizing horses, and although some success has been claimed its use is not advocated.
2. Gastric lavage (p. 23) should be undertaken, although in view of the long latent period it is unlikely to be productive.
3. Atropinisation should be carried out during phase 1, as many of the features may be due to the effects of muscarine. Atropine sulphate (2 mg) should be given intravenously followed by 1 mg every 10 minutes till features of atropinisation are evident.
4. Intensive supportive therapy (p. 18) is required to correct dehydration, severe acidosis, low blood calcium, potassium, sugar and hyperpyrexia.
5. In severe poisoning, a regimen for acute liver failure may be required, and exchange transfusion may be of value.
6. Haemodialysis may prevent hepatic coma if undertaken within 48 hours of ingestion. The toxins are of low molecular weight and may be diffusible, but they are firmly bound to proteins some 36 hours after ingestion.

AMANITA MUSCARIA—FLY AGARIC

This has a scarlet cap covered with white warts, and white gills on the stem. Because it looks poisonous, it is not commonly eaten. It has a reputation for being deadly but it is very much less toxic than *A. phalloides*.

AMANITA PANTHERINA—PANTHER CAP

This is occasionally mistaken for the edible species, the True Blusher, which it resembles. They may however be distinguished as when cut or broken the True Blusher's flesh becomes suffused with a pink or reddish colour; the Panther Cap remains white.

Both *A. muscaria* and *A. pantherina* have muscarine derivatives as their chief toxin. These are powerful stimulants of the parasympathetic nervous system. In contrast to *A. phalloides*, symptoms appear within one or two hours after ingestion. The features of poisoning closely resemble those produced by insecticides which act by inhibition of cholinesterase (p. 173). Symptoms include nausea, vomiting, diarrhoea, which may be associated with rice water motions, and severe abdominal cramp. Pallor, excessive salivation, slow pulse, bronchorrhoea and the constriction of the bronchioles are also features. Subsequent collapse, severe dehydration, and circulatory and respiratory failure may ensue. Features similar to intoxication, delirium or hallucinations may all occur.

Treatment

1. Gastric aspiration and lavage are essential (p. 23).
2. Intensive supportive therapy with careful biochemical control (p. 18).
3. Repeated doses of atropine sulphate to ensure adequate atropinisation are indicated in moderate or severe poisoning (p. 174).

Very careful observation is essential because on rare occasions symptoms and signs may be due to atropine (p. 114) rather than muscarine, as at certain phases in the

TABLE VIII—POISONOUS PLANTS, SHRUBS AND TREES

A comprehensive work such as British Poisonous Plants, H.M. Stationery Office 1954, should be consulted.   The following summary is given for the species which are most commonly regarded as poisonous.

Name	Poisonous part	Clinical features	Treatment
ACONITE (Monkshood)	All parts but chiefly seeds and roots.	Tingling and burning of mouth and skin. Nausea, vomiting, diarrhoea, agitation, collapse, convulsions.	1. Symptomatic. 2. Atropine sulphate (2 mg) intramuscularly if severe.
BERBERIS	Berries	Purging	Symptomatic.
BROOM	Poisonous only in very large amounts.	Similar to Laburnum but much less severe.	1. Gastric aspiration and lavage. 2. Symptomatic.
CHERRY	Stones if chewed and broken.	As for cyanide poisoning.	Page 65.
COTONEASTER	Berries NOT poisonous.	Nil.	Nil.
DAFFODIL	Bulb.	Nausea, vomiting, diarrhoea.	1. Gastric aspiration and lavage. 2. Symptomatic.
DEADLY NIGHTSHADE	All parts especially roots and berries. Very poisonous.	Atropinisation, excited, drowsy stupor.	1. Gastric lavage. 2. Artificial respiration. 3. Barbiturate. 4. Neostigmine 5 mg repeated at intervals.
ELDERBERRY	Leaves and bark.	As for cyanide poisoning.	Page 65.
HEMLOCK	'Seeds'.	Paralysis. Slow pulse. Dilated pupils. Rapid breathing and then respiratory failure.	1. Symptomatic. 2. Artificial respiration.
HOLLY	Berries	Nausea, vomiting, diarrhoea; mild sedation.	1. Gastric aspiration and lavage. 2. Symptomatic.
HYDRANGEA	All parts.	As for cyanide poisoning.	Page 65.

TABLE VIII.—continued

Name	Poisonous part	Clinical features	Treatment
LABURNUM	All parts, but when ripe, poison concentrated in seeds, pods and leaves. Next to the yew, is Britain's most poisonous tree.	Burning in mouth, nausea, intractable vomiting, diarrhoea, exhaustion, collapse. Delirium, convulsions and coma.	1. Gastric aspiration and lavage. 2. Symptomatic.
LUPIN	Seeds, but other parts to lesser extent.	Depression of respiration, paralysis, convulsions, collapse.	1. Gastric aspiration and lavage. 2. Symptomatic.
MARIHUANA	Leaves.	Stimulation of senses. Hallucinations, ataxia, blurred vision, diminished consciousness.	1. Gastric aspiration and lavage if ingested. 2. Symptomatic.
MISTLETOE	Berries but also all parts.	Nausea, vomiting, diarrhoea. Slow pulse.	1. Gastric aspiration and lavage. 2. As for digitalis (p. 135).
NARCISSUS	Bulbs.	Nausea, vomiting, diarrhoea.	Symptomatic.
NASTURTIUM	Seeds NOT poisonous.	Nil.	Nil.
SWEET PEA	NOT poisonous.	Nil.	Nil.
YEW	All parts, but especially the seeds. Britain's most poisonous tree.	Vomiting, abdominal colic, diarrhoea, paralysis, circulatory failure. Convulsions. Death often within five minutes.	An acute emergency. 1. Wash out stomach. 2. Pentothal for convulsions. 3. Artificial respiration.

growth of these mushrooms the predominant toxin produced may be atropine rather than muscarine.

REFERENCES

Poisonous Fungi, Plants, Shrubs and Trees
1 Hardin, J. W. and Arena, J. M. (1973). *Human Poisoning fron Native and Cultivated Plants*. North Carolina: Duke University Press.
2 Pamela, M. (1967). *Poisonous Plants and Fungi*. London: Blandford Press.

CHAPTER 25

DRUG ADDICTION

Drug addiction, or to use the World Health Organization term, drug dependence, is increasing amongst young people in Britain. Many adolescents, however, experiment with drugs but never become addicted. Acute overdosage occurs not only in the experimenter with drugs of dependence but also in the fully initiated. This is especially likely to occur when adulterated or unrefined preparations of these drugs are taken, for although the impurities usually render the substance less potent, on occasion the opposite obtains. In addition, as a result of rapidly developing tolerance to most drugs of addiction, the addict may become uncertain about his required dosage.

A recent trend in adolescent drug abuse in Britain is for a variety of drugs or substances to be taken rather than adhering to one drug. For example, when recent legislation made heroin more difficult to obtain, heroin addicts readily substituted other substances such as amphetamines, barbiturates or methaqualone intravenously. These drugs have totally different pharmacological effects from diamorphine and so these developments must raise some doubts about conventional concepts of drug dependence. The pleasure in the preparation of the injection, the cult of the needle and the satisfaction of the 'fix' must all play a part.

The drugs which commonly produce addiction can be loosely divided into three main groups: stimulants, depressants and those distorting the senses.

The Stimulants

The stimulants comprise the amphetamine group of drugs but also include sympathomimetic drugs such as ephedrine and methyl phenidate (Ritalin). In junkie parlance they are known as black bombers, purple hearts, French blues, Dex, pep pills and 'sweets'. Tolerance develops slowly but is often acquired to massive doses, e.g. 50 or more 5 mg dexedrine tablets at a time.

Clinical Features

In addicts these are both physical and psychological.

CENTRAL NERVOUS SYSTEM. Elation, excitability, aggression and talkativeness with a tendency to converse in junkie slang. These features are referred to by the junkie as the 'buzz' or being 'turned on'. Other common effects are delusions of persecution (the 'Noia'), hallucinations of being chased, often by the police (the 'Horrors') and excessive fatigue on Monday. Athetosis and repetitive 'head banging' may occur in chronic addiction.

GASTROINTESTINAL SYSTEM. Dryness of the mouth, ulcers of the buccal mucosa and anorexia with weight loss.

SKIN. Facial acne is common and in addition there is a rather characteristic erythema of the face.

URINE. Amphetamines give an orange colour when methyl orange is added to urine containing these drugs. This may be used as a reliable screening test for addiction, as a negative result indicates that the patient has taken less than 15 mg amphetamine.

Some addicts (meth-heads) still contrive to administer amphetamines (methylamphetamine-Methedrine) to themselves by intravenous injection. This however is now less common in Britain as a result of controls which have made this drug preparation available only in hospital.

Withdrawal Effects

The effects of acute overdosage and their treatment have been described (p. 110). These drugs may be stopped abruptly without fear of physical withdrawal features but psychological effects, which are often claimed to be minimal, are in fact quite common and usually take the form of severe depression and agitation.

The Depressants

The depressant drugs may be subdivided into hypnotics and narcotics.

HYPNOTICS

The chief hypnotics are barbiturates ('sleepers', 'goof balls') and Mandrax (methaqualone and diphenhydramine, 'mandies', p. 99). Tolerance develops rapidly. A small but significant number of addicts take the oral preparations of these drugs by injection. Difficulty is experienced in dissolving the contents of the tablets or capsules in water. Both oral barbiturates and Mandrax are strongly alkaline in solution, hence unless the injection technique is good the slightest leak may produce tissue necrosis. Digital gangrene may be induced by faulty injection into an artery.

Clinical Features

CENTRAL NERVOUS SYSTEM. Elation due to removal of inhibitions leading to confusion. Dilated pupils in the early stages. Nystagmus. Incoordination and later unconsciousness. With Mandrax, hypertonicity and hyper-reflexia may be prominent.

DIAGNOSIS. Barbiturate and methaqualone may be measured in both plasma and urine (p. 15).

Withdrawal Effects

The effects of acute overdosage of these substances and their management have been discussed (p. 48 and 99). About 24 hours after stopping the drug in a dependent patient withdrawal effects may occur. These include marked disturbance of sleep, anxiety, involuntary movements which may progress to convulsions and a state closely resembling delirium tremens.

NARCOTICS

The main narcotic drug is heroin (Horse, H). Methadone (Physeptone), cocaine and morphine are also in this group. Since recent legislation was introduced in Britain to provide strict control of supplies of diamorphine, the illicit trade in heroin has increased. Hence more adulterated preparations are being used by addicts; aspirin, lactose and quinine are often added. The route of administration is by subcutaneous injection ('skin popping') or intravenous injection ('mainlining'). A recent fashion probably to avoid detection by the authorities or because the more accessible veins are thrombosed, is to inject into the venous plexus under the tongue, in the rectum or in the vagina. Very rarely in older subjects heroin may be taken by mouth or as snuff as may cocaine ('snorkling'). Tolerance develops rapidly irrespective of the route of administration and large doses may be required by addicts to obtain the desired effect.

Clinical Features

CENTRAL NERVOUS SYSTEM. Pin-point pupils, which may dilate with nalorphine but this does not always happen in dependent subjects and so it is not a reliable diagnostic test. Transitory elation leading to anxiety and restlessness. Loss of libido. Totally unreliable and usually a convincing liar. Marked tendency to converse in junkie jargon.

GASTROINTESTINAL SYSTEM. Marked anorexia, constipation and severe weight loss. Icterus often due to serum jaundice from sharing syringes.

RESPIRATORY SYSTEM. A mysterious condition known as "allergic lung" may occur. The cause is uncertain. It is not a true allergy to heroin, but may be a reaction to an adulterant.

SKIN. Dirty and unkempt. Abscesses, bruises and septic thrombophlebitis at injection sites on the back of hands or cubital fossae. The dorsa of the hands may be brawny and swollen.

LABORATORY FINDINGS. A number of addicts may be Australia antigen positive. Precautions should be taken until

N

the result of this test is known.

Withdrawal Effects

It should be remembered that the addict is desperate to the point of distraction for the next injection ('fix') not so much to experience the transient euphoria, but rather to avoid the let down effects. He will, therefore, be extremely worried lest his injection kit ('gear') is removed or lost and he is unlikely to conceal the fact that he is 'hooked'. On the contrary he may give a highly coloured and exaggerated account of the severity of his addiction, showing his 'heroin tattooed' arm and demanding another injection. Withdrawal features, the torture which the addict knows can be prevented by another 'fix' include in the early stages:

Running nose and eyes, constant sneezing, gooseflesh, perspiration, vague aches and pains and dilated pupils.
Anxiety, restlessness and aggression are common.

The later 'cold turkey' stage is featured by:

Nausea, vomiting, abdominal pain, diarrhoea, limb cramps, sleeplessness, further agitation leading to collapse.

Prognosis

A large number of regular users of heroin die before the age of thirty. The cause of death may be septicaemia, bacterial endocarditis, tetanus, jaundice or acute overdosage. Addicts may develop a curious 'sensitivity' reaction which causes pulmonary oedema and death.

Treatment

It is illegal, unless he is specially licenced, for a doctor to prescribe heroin for an addict as defined under the Misuse of Drugs Act, 1971, Notification of and Supply to Addicts Regulations, 1973. A doctor in a casualty department confronted by a heroin addict is prevented by law from administering heroin. He should take the following steps:

1. If considered necessary to prevent withdrawal features, methadone (Physeptone) 10-20 mg in an orange drink should be given. In this way the dosage is readily concealed from the addict. The dose may be repeated in one to two hours. This will control symptoms for 12 hours.

2. The addict should be informed of the hospital where facilities for treating heroin addicts are available and given strong encouragement to attend such a hospital.

3. It is a statutory duty under the above Act to notify the addict to the Home Office. The regulations seek to avoid repetition of notification.
Information as to whether a patient has been notified may be obtained by telephoning the Home Office 01 799 3488, extensions 135 or 271. The hospital at which the addict is supposed to be attending can be determined, as can other details.

4. The 'allergic lung' must be dealt with energetically as it is a recognised cause of death in addicts. Intravenous injection of 200 mg hydrocortisone and frusemide 80 mg together with assisted ventilation should be given.

Drugs Causing Distortion of the Senses

Cannabis (Pot, Hash, Hemp, Weed, Marijuana, Reefers), Grass); d-lysergic acid diethylamide (L.S.D. 25, Sugar, Acid).

CANNABIS

Tolerance is not readily acquired. Smoking is almost the sole method of administration. Addiction in the true sense does not occur.

Clinical Features

The patient often looks lethargic with drooping eyelids and bloodshot conjunctivae.

CENTRAL NERVOUS SYSTEM. A dreamy feeling of benevolence and well being often with euphoria. Changes in perception of colours, shape and time, with improved appreciation of art and music. Libido may be increased; aggressive, irrational behaviour and rarely a toxic psychosis may be evident. Stupor ('stoned') may result from a large dose but there is no hangover effect. Cerebral atrophy has been reported, but the evidence is unconvincing. No proven effects on the foetus have been demonstrated.

GASTROINTESTINAL SYSTEM. Dry mouth. Appetite may be increased.

LONG TERM EFFECTS. It has not been determined yet whether or not lung cancer may be induced by cannabis smoking.

Withdrawal Effects

There is doubt as to whether cannabis should be classified as a drug of dependence for there are no physical effects of withdrawal and, apart from resentment, no psychic effects.

Treatment of Overdose

The principles of intensive supportive therapy (p. 18) should be followed but the patient is seldom other than drowsy and should be simply allowed to sleep off the effects.

L.S.D.

Any administration except by specially licenced practitioners is illegal. The dose required to produce psychotropic effects ('take a trip') is about 200 μg, but tolerance is readily acquired. It is usually taken orally on a lump of sugar, as a black market tablet or in the fashionable 'micro-dot' preparation.

Clinical Features

CENTRAL NERVOUS SYSTEM. Profound and terrifying emotional upsets may be experienced which may reach beyond the control of the 'guide', i.e. the one individual in the group who has not 'taken a trip'. There is distortion of sound and colour. Depersonalisation and dissociation which can last for hours or days may occur and visual, auditory and tactile hallucinations are common. Experiences of the past may be relived (this is the action of the drug employed by psychiatrists in treating severe obsessional and other neurotic states). A toxic psychosis lasting on occasion for months may be induced.

FLASHBACK PHENOMENON. This may occur many months after 'taking a trip' and the person experiences a recurrence of the emotional and psychological aspects of the previous 'L.S.D. trip'. Very abnormal behaviour may be present such as a belief in being able to fly. The time elapsed since the previous 'trip' may be so long that the association with L.S.D. may be missed.

REPRODUCTIVE SYSTEM. Although not conclusive there is now good evidence to suggest that L.S.D. has an adverse effect on the chromosomes and on the foetus.

Withdrawal Effects

No physical effects are observed. This substance is usually employed intermittently and most addicts can readily wait till circumstances are propitious for the next 'trip'.

Treatment of Overdose

Large doses of chlorpromazine—200 mg intramuscularly repeated in half an hour and thereafter as necessary, are required to combat the acute effects.

CHAPTER 26

PREVENTION OF ACUTE POISONING

Eighty per cent of admissions of poisoned adult patients are suffering from self-poisoning, a conscious, often impulsive act. Very few adults suffer from poisoning which is truly accidental. In children, however, most instances are accidental but in the age group 11-15 years self-poisoning may be encountered. Both in adults and in children a major predisposing factor is the ready availability of medicaments and household preparations. Doctors can make a very important contribution to the prevention of poisoning by accepting as their responsibility certain precautions which should be taken both by them and by their patients[1].

The much repeated 'Lock up your Medicines' is perhaps becoming so familiar that it is losing its force. In the prevention of poisoning in children there is no substitute for keeping all medicines in a locked cupboard. 'All medicines' include iron tablets, salicylates, contraceptive pills and liniments, for these are the most common medicines taken by children.

Another important factor is that pharmaceutical firms often prepare tablets and capsules in a variety of attractive colours and shapes which are similar to many popular sweets and therefore very attractive to children. This danger is increased by parents who, often with the best intentions, encourage their children to take medicines by suggesting that the tablets are, in fact, sweets. It would be a valuable advance in preventive medicine if drug houses could find it possible to promote their products in a less colourful way! Many potent and dangerous drugs are now dispensed as pleasant elixirs and syrups with an increased danger of overdosage in the unwitting toddler or the careless adult.

Poisoning by bleach and household preparations is also common in children under the age of 5 years and will continue to be so long as these articles are stored at floor level and available to the inquisitive toddler.

In adults with the impulsive conscious element in self-poisoning, availability of drugs is also very important. Hoarding of drugs, either wilfully or thoughtlessly, is extremely common. The doctor should play his part in prevention of self-poisoning by making sure that large amounts of sedative and antidepressant drugs are not available. He should, therefore, prescribe only minimum quantities of drugs for certain individuals and routinely inspect home medicine cupboards to ensure that drugs not in current use have been disposed of and are not stored.

In the prevention of self-poisoning, which is so often an unstated appeal for help, the doctor should in a number of instances anticipate the self-poisoning act and take due notice of the distress which precipitates the episode. Appropriate measures should be taken to deal with the situation before the patient has to indulge in the manipulative act of taking an overdose.

The provision of drug containers which toddlers find difficult or impossible to open is to be encouraged[2]. The wrapping of individual tablets in foil is also a notable safety measure. This is a legal requirement in the United States, but in the United Kingdom legislation is sadly lacking.

Frequently, dangerous chemicals, such as weed-killers and turpentine are stored in the home or garden in bottles which previously contained lemonade or beer and which remain so labelled. This accounts for instances of accidental poisoning in both adults and children. The remedy is obvious, but all too often omitted.

Acute accidental poisoning in industry is uncommon in Britain. For this much credit must be given to legislation which lays down stringent conditions regarding the storage, transport and use of many potentially poisonous substances. The introduction of automatic techniques has provided a means whereby essential processing, using noxious substances can be done mechanically and without exposing individuals to the risk of poisoning. Many of these improvements have been introduced on the initiative of Industrial Medical Officers.

Due to the introduction of numerous potent drugs the risk of iatrogenic poisoning by inappropriate treatment is now very real. Salicylate poisoning in children may also be iatrogenic, particularly if the child is dehydrated and is not given adequate fluids. The dosage schedule in any event should not exceed 60 mg per year of life, five times a day. This regimen should not be continued for longer than two days.

At various times attempts have been made to incorporate in the sedative, hypnotic or antidepressant tablet, another substance which it was thought might lessen the toxic effects in the event of an overdosage. Such 'built in' remedies are ipecac or an analeptic. In neither instance has the ingenious idea proved of practical value; in the former, because the amount of added ipecac required was too large, and in the latter because no analeptic drug could be found which would be sufficiently potent when taken by mouth.

The prevention of acute poisoning thus provides a challenge for all doctors.

REFERENCES

1 Matthew, H. (1972/73). *Prevent.*, **1**, 57.
2 Breault, H. J. (1974). *Clin. Toxicol.*, **7**, 91.

INDEX

Accidental poisoning, incidence, 4, 44.
  prevention, 192
Acetaminophen, 76.
Aconite, 181.
Activated charcoal, 23.
Adder bite, 165.
Age, choice of poison, 7.
Alcohol, associated with self-poisoning, 8.
  poisoning by ethyl, 129.
  poisoning by methyl, 128.
Allegron, 81
Allobarbitone, duration of action, 49.
Amitryptyline, 81.
Amphetamine, forced acid diuresis, 35, 111.
  measurement in urine and blood, 110.
  tolerance to, 109, 184.
  toxic dose, 109.
  treatment, 110.
Amylobarbitone, duration of action, 49.
Analeptic drugs, adverse effects, 28.
  in respiratory failure, 20.
Antabuse, 131.
  reaction with alcohol, 132.
Antibiotic poisoning, 150.
Antibiotics, prophylactic use, 29.
Anticoagulants, 149.
Antidepressant drugs, clinical features of poisoning, 82.
  pharmacology, 81.
  prognosis in poisoning, 83.
  physostigmine in treatment, 83.
  treatment of poisoning, 82.
Antidotes, infrequently available, 2
  universal, 25.

Antihistamines, 147.
Antivenins, 165.
Antivenum in adder bite, 165.
Apomorphine, 23.
Aramine, in shock, 21.
Arsenic, 119.
Arvynol, 102.
Atropine poisoning, clinical features, 114.
  from various fruits and berries, 181.
  treatment, 114.
Aventyl, 81.

BAL, 125.
Barbitone, duration of action, 49.
Barbiturate poisoning, assessment of severity, 50.
  availability of drugs, 48.
  barbitone and dialysis, 55.
  barbiturate metabolites, 50.
  blisters, 12, 53.
  blood levels, 19, 33, 50.
    and assessment, 50.
  cardiovascular system, 52.
  central nervous system, 51.
  clinical features, 51.
  combination of drugs, 50.
  complications from short acting, 48.
  chemical estimation, 15.
  diagnosis, 12, 48.
  effects on skin, 53.
  fallacies in assessment, 48, 50.
  forced diuresis, 33, 38, 54.
  gastrointestinal system, 53.
  haemodialysis, 38, 41, 54.
  hypothermia, 52.
  incidence, 48.

195

Barbiturate poisoning–*contd.*
  peritoneal dialysis, 36, 38.
  phenobarbitone and dialysis, 38, 55.
  phenobarbitone blood levels, 19.
  removal of drug from body, 38, 54.
  renal failure, 53.
  respiratory system, 52.
  shock, 21, 52.
  treatment, 54.
Barbiturates, long acting, 49.
  medium acting, 49.
  short acting, 49.
Belladonna alkaloids, 113.
Bemegride, 28.
  and barbiturate estimation, 29.
  and glutethimide estimation, 29.
Benzedrine, 109.
Benzene, 67.
Benzodiazepins, 93.
Benzol, 67.
Berberis, 181.
Biguanides, 153.
Black Widow spider, 166.
Bladder catheterisation, contra-indicated, 29.
  in severe poisoning, 29.
Bleaches, 156, 157.
Blindness, in methyl alcohol poisoning, 128, 129.
  in quinine poisoning, 136.
Blood levels, in habituation, 16, 19.
  in tolerance, 16, 19.
Bromides, 151.
Broom, 181.
Brown recluse spider, 167.
Bullae, in barbiturate poisoning, 12, 53.
  in carbon monoxide poisoning, 12, 59.
  in glutethimide poisoning, 12.
  in tricyclic antidepressants, 12.
  treatment, 27.

Butobarbitone, duration of action, 49.

Calomel, 122.
Camcolit, 86.
Carbamates, 94.
Carbon monoxide poisoning, arrhythmias, 59.
  bullae, 12, 59.
  cardiovascular system, 59.
  central nervous system, 58.
  clinical features, 58.
  diagnosis, 13, 58.
  effects of age, 58.
  effects on cerebral tissue, 57, 58.
  effects on skin, 59.
  elderly patients, 58.
  5 per cent carbon dioxide in treatment, 60.
  gastrointestinal system, 59.
  high mortality, 56.
  hyperbaric oxygen, 61.
  myocardial damage, 58, 59.
  oxygen, 60.
  properties of gas, 57.
  respiratory system, 59.
  sequelae of damage, 57.
  treatment, 60.
    of cerebral oedema, 60.
Carbon tetrachloride, 64.
Cheese, monoamine oxidase inhibitors, reactions with, 84.
Cherry, 181.
Chloral hydrate, 101.
Chlorate, 157.
Chlordiazepoxide, 93.
Cocktail diuresis, 34.
Codeine, 138.
Concordin, 81.
Consciousness, level of and pupils, 19.
  limb reflexes and level, 19.
  loss of, grading, 18.
Contraceptive pill, 150.

Corrosive sublimate, 122.
Cotoneaster, 181.
Cresol, 158.
Cyanide poisoning, 65.
Cyclobarbitone, duration of action, 49.
Cycloserine, 150.
Cysteamine in Paracetamol Poisoning, 76, 78.

Daffodil, 181.
Darvon, 140.
Deadly nightshade, 181.
Death cap mushroom, 178.
Dehydration, treatment, 27.
Delirium tremens, 130.
Depronal, 141.
Desferrioxamine, in iron poisoning, 119.
Desipramine, 81.
Detergents, 161.
Dexamphetamine sulphate, 109, 184.
Dexedrine, 109, 184.
Diagnosis of poisoning, 12.
Dial, duration of action, 49.
Dialysis, use in various poisonings, 38.
Diazepam, 93, 108.
Dichlorphenazone, 101.
Digitalis, in poisoning by phenothiazines, 91.
Digitalis poisoning, 134.
Dihydrocodeine, 138, 146.
Dimercaprol, in poisoning by metals, 121, 123, 125.
Dinitro-ortho-cresol, 171.
Dinitro-phenol, 171.
Diphenoxylate, 143.
Dipipanone, 138.
Di-Quat, 175.
Distalgesic, 141.
Disulfiram, 131.
Doloxene, 141.
Doloxytal, 141.

Doriden, 97.
Doxepin, 81.
Drug addiction, adolescent abuse, 184.
    amphetamines, 184.
    bacterial endocarditis, 188.
    barbiturates, 186.
    cannabis, 189.
    depersonalisation, 190.
    depressants, 186.
    distortion of senses, 189.
    d-lysergic acid diethylamide, 189 190.
    ephedrine, 184.
    hemp, 189.
    heroin, 187.
    hypnotics, 186.
    intravenous administration, 185, 186, 187.
    jaundice, 187.
    L.S.D., 190.
    Mandrax, 186.
    marijuana, 189.
    methaqualone, 186.
    methadone, 189.
    methedrine, 185.
    methyl orange test, 185.
    nalorphine test, 187.
    narcotics, 187.
    notification of addicts, 188.
    Physeptone, 189.
    septicaemia, 188.
    skin, 185, 187.
    stimulants, 184.
    supply to addicts, 188.
    tolerance, 184.
    treatment, 188, 190, 191.
    withdrawal effects, 185, 186, 188, 190, 191.
Drug dependence. See Drug addiction.

Elderberry, 181.
Emergency measures in treatment, 19.

Emesis, induction of, 22.
Emetic drugs, 23.
Ephedrine, 112, 184.
Ethchlorvynol, 102.
Ethyl alcohol, 129.
in treatment of methyl alcohol poisoning, 129.
Epanutin, 105.
Equanil, 94.
Errors in treatment, analeptic therapy, 28.
bemegride, 28.
bladder catheterisation, 29.
Megimide, 28.
prophylactic antibiotics, 29.
Ethinamate, 94, 95.
Evipan, duration of action, 49.

Fenfluramine, 111.
Fire extinguishers, 64.
Forced acid diuresis, ammonium chloride, 35.
contraindications, 33.
in amphetamine poisoning, 35, 110.
in quinine poisoning, 35, 137.
technique, 35.
Forced alkaline diuresis, 35.
contraindications, 33.
Forced diuresis, for salicylate poisoning, 34.
contraindications, 33.
Fructose in treatment of ethyl alcohol poisoning, 130.
Frusemide, in forced alkaline diuresis, 35.
in noxious gas poisoning, 30.
Funnel web spider, 166.

Gastric aspiration and lavage, aspiration of vomitus, 23.
conscious level, 23.
contraindications, 22.
endotracheal intubation, 23.
equipment, 24.

Gastric aspiration and lavage—contd.
lavage fluid, ordinary, 24.
special circumstances, 26.
position of patient, 24.
substances left in stomach, 26.
time interval since ingestion, 23.
Glutethimide poisoning, 97.
bullae, 12.
clinical features, 97.
increased intracranial pressure, 98.
pharmacology, 97.
plasma levels, 98.
prognosis, 99.
treatment, 98.
Gold, 121.

Haemodialysis, in treatment, 38, 39, 40, 41.
Hemlock, 181.
Herbicides, 171.
Heroin addiction, clinical features, 187.
notification, 189.
prognosis, 188.
treatment, 188.
withdrawal effects, 188.
Heroin poisoning, 138.
Hexobarbitone, duration of action, 49.
Holly, 181.
Homatropine, 114.
Hydantoin compounds, 105.
Hydrangea, 181.
Hydrocortisone, in hypothermia, 28.
in noxious gas poisoning, 30.
in shock, 22.
Hyperbaric oxygen, cerebrovascular resistance, 61.
in carbon monoxide poisoning, 61.
portable chamber, 62.
Hypothermia, 27, 52, 91.

Identification of poison, chemical identification of common drugs, 14.
code letter and number, 13.
Hefferrens method, 14.
lack of importance, 13.
McArdle's method, 14.
visual, 13.
Imipramine poisoning, 81.
Insect bites, 166.
Insecticides, 171.
Intensive supportive therapy, 18.
frequency of use, 30.
Ipecacuanha, Syrup of, 23.
Iron poisoning, 117.
clinical features, 117.
desferrioxamine, 119.
treatment, 118.
Isoprenaline, 112.
Isoproterenol, 112.

Jellyfish, 169.

Kelocyanor, in cyanide poisoning, 66.
Kerosene poisoning, 62.
gastric aspiration and lavage, 22, 63.

L.S.D., clinical features, 190.
treatment of overdose, 191.
withdrawal effects, 191.
Laroxyl, 81.
Laburnum, 182.
Lead poisoning, 123.
level in blood, 124.
treatment, 125.
urinary output, 125.
Lethidrone, 112.
Librium, 93.
Lithium, 39, 86.
Lomotil, 143.
Luminal, duration of action, 49
Lupin, 182.
Lysol, 12, 158.

Malayan Pit Viper, 164.

Malathion, 171, 173.
Mandrax poisoning, 99.
addiction, 186.
Mannitol, in carbon monoxide poisoning, 60.
in forced alkaline osmotic diuresis, 35.
Marihuana, addiction, 189.
plant, 182.
Matches, poisonous varieties, 161.
Medinal, duration of action, 49.
Megimide, 28.
Mepavlon, 94.
Meprobamate, 94.
Mercury, 122.
Mesontoin, 106.
Metaldehyde, 161.
Metallic poisoning, 117.
Metaraminol in shock, 21.
Methaemoglobinaemia, 158.
Methanol, 128.
Methaqualone, 99, 186.
Methoin, 106.
Methyl alcohol, 128.
Methyl amphetamine, addiction, 185.
effects, 110, 185.
Methylpentynol carbamate, 95,102.
Miscellaneous organic solvents, 67.
Miltown, 94.
Mistletoe, 182.
Mogadon, 93, 103.
Monoamine oxidase inhibitors, clinical features of poisoning 84.
interaction with cheese, 84.
interaction with drugs, 84, 85.
interaction with tyramine, 84.
treatment of interaction, 86.
treatment of poisoning, 85.
Morphine, 138.
Mushroom poisoning, 178.
Amanita muscaria, 180.
Amanita pantherina, 180.
Amanita phalloides, 178, 180.

Mushrooms, poisonous species, 178.
Mysoline, 106.

Nalorphine, eye test in addicts, 187.
  in opiate poisoning, 139.
Naloxone, 139, 142, 144.
Naphthalene, 160.
Narcissus, 182.
Nasturtium, 182.
Nembutal, duration of action, 49.
Nikethimide, 20, 28.
Nitrazepam, 93, 103.
Non-barbiturate anticonvulsants, 105.
Non-barbiturate hypnotics, dependence, 97.
  safety, 97.
Nortriptyline, 81.
Noxious gas poisoning, 56.
Nursing care in acute poisoning, 25.

Oblivon C, 94, 102.
Opium alkaloids, 138.
Oral diuretics, 146.
Oral hypoglycaemic agents, 153.
Organophosphorous compounds, 173.
  cholinesterase inhibition, 173.
  pralidoxime, 174.
  treatment, 174.
Ospolot, 107.
Oxalic acid, 26, 157.
Oxygen, in carbon monoxide poisoning, 60.
  in respiratory failure, 20.

Panadol, 76
Paracetamol, hepatic damage in, 76.
Paraldehyde, 106.
Paraffin, 62.
  gastric aspiration and lavage, 23, 63.
Paraquat, 175.

Parathion, 171, 173.
Penicillamine, in acute lead poisoning, 126.
Pentobarbitone, duration of action, 49.
Pentothal, duration of action, 49.
Peritoneal dialysis, added albumen, 37.
  basic principles, 36.
  complications, 41.
  correction of acid-base imbalance 36.
  correction of electrolyte imbalance, 37.
  dialysis fluid, 36.
  efficacy, 37.
  factors important, 36.
  in treatment, 36.
  procedure, 37.
  use of Impersol, 37.
Pertofran, 81.
Pethidine, 138.
Petroleum distillates, 62.
Phanodorm, duration of action, 49.
Phenacetin, 75.
Phenobarbitone poisoning, 48.
  blood level, 32.
  duration of action, 49.
  haemodialysis, 38.
  peritoneal dialysis, 36, 38.
Phenol poisoning, 12, 158.
Phenothiazine poisoning, 89.
  blood levels, 90.
  clinical features, 90.
  toxicological diagnosis, 91.
  treatment, 91.
Phenytoin, 105.
Phosphorus, 126.
Physostigmine Salicylate in poisoning with Antidepressant drugs, 83.
Placidyl, 102.
Poisons Information Service, centres, 10.
  telephone numbers, 11.

Potassium, in digitalis poisoning, 135.
in forced alkaline diuresis, 35.
Pralidoxime, available supplies, 174.
in organophosphorous poisoning 174.
Prevention of acute poisoning, 192.
Priadel, 86.
Primidone, 106.
Pro-Banthine, 115.
Propranolol, in poisoning with phenothiazines, 91.
Propantheline bromide, 115.
Propoxyphene, 140.
Protriptyline, 81.
Psychiatric disposal of patients, 46.
Psychiatric illness in poisoned patients, 46.
Psychiatric treatment, follow-up, 43.
Psychiatrist, self-poisoning and, 43.

Quaalude, 99.
Quinalbarbitone, duration of action 49.
Quinidine, 135.
Quinine, as abortifacient, 136.
Quinine, clinical features of poisoning, 136.
forced acid diuresis, 35, 137.
treatment of poisoning, 136.

Rauwolfia alkaloids, 91.
Reserpine, 91.
Respiratory failure, analeptic drugs in, 20.
artificial respiration, 20.
aspiration pneumonia, 20.
coramine, 20.
nikethimide, 20.
oxygen, 20.
tracheostomy, 21.
Water's canister, 20.
Wright's spirometer, 20.

Salicylate, biochemical estimation, 14.
Salicylate poisoning, 69.
absorption from skin, 69.
blood levels, 14, 70.
importance, 70.
clinical features, 71.
in children, 71.
cocktail diuresis, 34, 73.
complications, 72.
diagnosis, 12, 70.
forced alkaline diuresis, 35, 73.
contraindications, 33.
in children, 75.
precautions, 34.
technique, 35.
gastric aspiration and lavage, 72.
haemodialysis, 41, 74.
incidence, 69.
laboratory findings, 71, 72.
in adults, 71.
in children, 72.
peritoneal dialysis, 36, 74.
preparations used, 69.
severe dehydration, 71, 73.
therapeutic production, 69.
treatment, 72.
Trinder's method of quantification, 14.
Saroten, 81.
Scopolamine, 114.
Scorpions, 168.
Sea snake bite, 165.
Seconal, duration of action, 49.
Self-poisoning, alcohol and, 44.
anticipation of crisis, 44.
coal gas, 44.
definition, 4.
impulsiveness, 44.
incidence, 5, 44.
prevention, 192.
psychiatric assessment, 43.
resulting physical illness, 44.
role of psychiatrist, 44.
size of overdose, 45.

Sex ratio of poisoning, 7.
Shock, acidaemia, 21.
  Aramine, 21.
  dangers of intravenous infusions, 22.
  definition, 21.
  hydrocortisone, 22.
  mechanism in barbiturate poisoning, 21.
  metaraminol, 21.
  treatment, 21.
Sinequan, 81.
Snail bait, 161.
Snake bite, 163.
Sodium barbitone, duration of action, 49.
Sodium bicarbonate, in forced alkaline diuresis, 34, 35.
Sodium hypochlorite, 156.
Soneryl, duration of action, 49.
Special methods of treatment, 32.
  methods available, 33.
  recovery of drug, 32.
Spider bites, 166.
Sting rays, 168.
Suicidal poisoning incidence, 4.
Sulphonylureas, 154.
Sulthiame, 107.
Surmontil, 81.
Sweet pea, 182.

Telephone numbers, Information Service, 11.
Tepp, 171, 173.
Tertiary alcohols, 102.
Thallium, 151.

Thermometer, broken, 122.
Thiazides, 146.
Thiopentone, duration of action, 49.
Tofranil, 81.
Tracheostomy, time factor, 21.
Tranquilliser drugs, 89.
Triclofos, 101.
Tricloryl, 101.
Tricyclic poisoning, 81.
Trimipramine, 81.
Triptafen, 81.
Tryptizol, 81.
Turpentine, 161.

Universal antidote, 25.

Valium, 93, 108.
Valmid, 94.
Valmidate, 94.
Venomous animals, 165.
Venomous sea animals, 168.
Veronal, duration of action, 49.
Versene, in acute lead poisoning, 125.
Vipera berus, 165.

Weaver Fish, 169.
Welldorm, 101.
Withdrawal effects, barbiturate, 52.
  delirium tremens, 130.
  in drug addiction, 185, 186, 188, 190, 191.
Wright's spirometer, 20.

Yew, 182.